Crystal massage for everyone

Michael Gienger
& Ulrich Metz

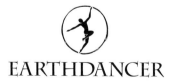

EARTHDANCER

A FINDHORN PRESS IMPRINT

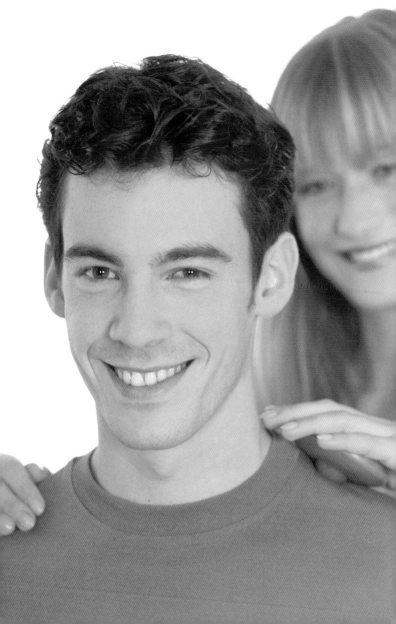

Contents

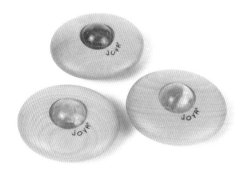

Everyone Can Massage!

Massage is a very enjoyable experience! It is simply a great pleasure to be massaged by sensitive, empathetic hands – and it is an equal pleasure to bring wellbeing to another through a good massage. Touching (Arabic 'massa' = 'to touch') is a basic human need, and yet it is so often neglected! Let's be honest, how many massages do you allow yourself per week? Or should we ask, 'per month' or 'per year'? And how many massages are still owed to you by your partner? Massage probably counts among the things most frequently promised and then forgotten in relationships...

But what is it *really* that dissuades us from giving each other pleasure with loving and attentive massage? Why do we not make the space and time for this kind of caring and closeness, and even relief from tension and pain?

In essence there are usually three factors that keep us from massaging. The first is the fear that we don't know how to do it properly, that we don't know how to massage certain parts of the body in the right way (apart from the shoulders, it is not always clear how to go about it); we feel uncertain. Second, there is the effort involved in giving a massage, as the hands, and particularly the thumbs, will quickly start to hurt if one is not used to massaging. Third, there is the time and preparation required. The room has to be cleared first, and has to be heated and prepared. Then there is likely to be no proper massage table to hand, and the floor is too hard, the bed too soft... By the time everything has been optimally prepared, the impulse and the energy have dissipated; so we let go, and decide maybe to watch television together, which is, well, quite pleasant too...

So, the good intention is there, but seeing it through is chock full of uncertainties or is just a little too much effort.

It need not be so! Ulrich Metz has created a smart little massage tool called the Joya® Massage Roller; it is so simple to use that you will soon overcome your uncertainties about massage. It really is true – anyone can carry out a massage with this tool! The roller reduces the strain on the hands and fingers making massaging easier. It is also universally applicable – you don't need to clear up half the living room to make space; you can massage anywhere you happen to be! Whether at home, at work, on holiday, or travelling, whether clothed or unclothed, it makes no difference; the Joya® Massage Roller brings wellbeing in no time at all.

The very presence of this simple but aesthetically pleasing roller will motivate you to have a go at massaging. If the roller is lying around in the living room, it will encourage you to do something pleasurable for another, especially if your partner is complaining about a tension headache or tired legs. If it is lying around in the bedroom, you can use it as an aid for sleeplessness, as well as for creating a pleasurable evening for two. And it should definitely be included in your luggage to help with minor complaints when travelling.

In the four years that I have been familiarising myself with the Joya® Massage Roller, I have given far more brief, 'in between' massages – both to myself and to others – than in the entire preceding twenty years! Thanks to several courses in massage, uncertainty was never my main obstacle, but instead I felt put off by having to prepare. All that simply disappears with Joya® massage.

With this little booklet, we cordially invite you to try out Joya® massage. You will see that massaging really is easy!

Tübingen, Summer 2008
Michael Gienger

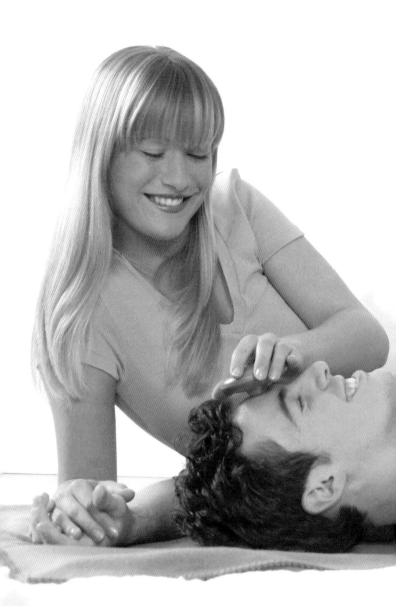

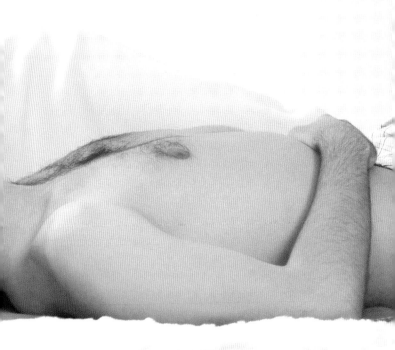

Massage is Easy!

Massage is Easy!

The Joya® Massage Roller

The Joya® massage roller consists of two components – the wooden hand-piece* and a freely rotating crystal sphere. Together they make it possible to give a massage while remaining relaxed, a great benefit for the masseur. For the recipient, the rolling motion of the sphere feels really good on the skin and less pressure needs to be applied. Defensive tenseness is avoided, allowing the massage to be much more effective. Another plus is that the crystal spheres can be exchanged and therefore adapted to the purpose of the massage. Each crystal sphere brings its own special crystal healing properties (see page 112), which can support, guide and intensify the massage.

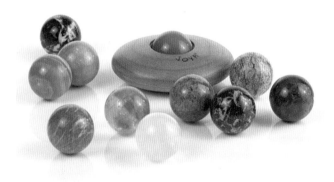

* Hand-pieces made of mineral composite substances, and therefore easy to disinfect, can be supplied for therapeutic practices, see page 126.

Choosing a Hand-piece

Before carrying out a Joya® massage, (or when purchasing a roller), choose a hand-piece that feels right to you. Hold and feel a few different ones to get a sense of each type of wood; even though identical in shape, each will feel different. If chosen in this way, it will be your own personal perception that selects your hand-piece.

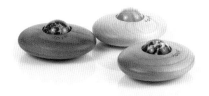

Hand-pieces made of different types of wood:
Walnut, Birch and Cherry (left to right).

Each type of wood has its own individual characteristics, which become visible with closer inspection, and can be sensed during the massage:

Light-coloured hand-pieces are made of **Birch**, which bestows dexterity and mobility. It encourages lightness and mobility of the fingers during a massage. As a water-loving tree, Birch supports circulation of the body fluids and heightened perception in the person being treated.

Reddish-brown hand-pieces are made of **Cherry**, which fortifies warm-heartedness and attentive care, as well as the ability to feel and be empathetic. For the person being treated, Cherry supports relaxation and letting go, and therefore deepens the effects of a massage.

Dark brown hand-pieces are made of **Walnut**, which combines concentration and discipline with aesthetics and harmony. In this way, Walnut enhances clear perception and sensitivity. For the person being treated, Walnut brings wellbeing, inner peace, balance and mental stability.

Choosing a Crystal Sphere

A crystal sphere can be chosen intuitively, by you or by the person being treated. If you are choosing for the person receiving the Joya® massage, inwardly adapt yourself to that person by asking yourself, 'What would be good for him or her?'; then choose the crystal sphere that *immediately* 'speaks' to you, in that first second, which may not necessarily be the one you 'like' most! The person being treated can proceed in the same way when choosing their own crystal sphere, or simply ask them to close their eyes and choose the sphere 'blind'. Closed eyes make it easier for the body to sense and signal what would be good for it.

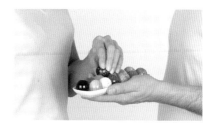

Intuitive choice of crystal sphere

When acquiring the Joya® massage roller and a selection of crystal spheres, it is of course essential to consider the effects and inherent qualities of the crystals. Detailed crystal information can be found in the crystal 'portraits' beginning on page 112.

Assembling the Roller

The wooden hand-piece and the chosen crystal sphere are put together by gently pressing the sphere into the opening – that's all you have to do to make the roller ready for use. The Teflon ring around the opening holds the sphere in place so that it cannot fall out, but also leaves it free to move and roll unrestricted. Use the little suction cap (gem remover) to remove the sphere again and to exchange it for another.

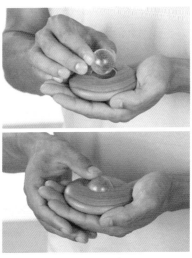

Assembling the
Joya® Massage Roller

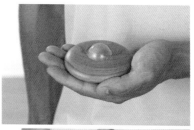

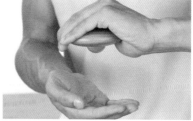

The sphere is held in place,
but is still completely mobile.

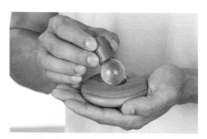

Using the suction cap (gem remover)
to remove the sphere

Space and Peace

The Joya® massage roller is now ready for use, and you can begin the massage. As already mentioned in the Introduction, a Joya® massage can be done anywhere. Loosen up your own tense shoulders at the office, or do something nice for a colleague. Offer your loved ones at home an enjoyable experience with an extensive massage. Treat back complaints during travelling. The location is secondary. While a quiet, protected space is always more pleasant and comfortable, the Joya® massage roller has proved itself particularly useful in situations where such a space is *not* available. Simply create that peace within yourself by adopting a relaxed position, breathing out consciously a few times (to help loosen tension), focussing, and then mentally 'setting aside' anything that might interfere (all that can wait!). You can then invite your massage partner into this 'peaceful space' you have created.

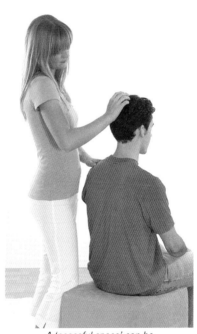

A 'peaceful space' can be created anywhere.

Protection

The closeness and touching that occurs during a massage favour an exchange of energies between the two persons involved. (The surroundings may also have a stronger general effect through this opening up and relaxing.) This type of energy exchange is not intentional. A massage promotes the recipient's own energy flow through touch; foreign energies absorbed during a massage, however, can be disturbing and interfering. You can be especially susceptible to energy exchange when you do not have a massage room available or if you are giving a short massage while out and about somewhere; it is therefore important to pay attention to good energetic protection.

Protection can be built up by visualizing (for example) a flame of violet light around yourself and your massage partner. Just conjure up the deep violet colour of a beautiful amethyst around yourself and then envelop the other person in it too. Visualizing violet light has a purifying, clearing and protecting effect.

A further possibility for protection consists of imagining a horizontal figure-of-eight made of light, which lies around you and the other person, so that each of you is placed in one of the two loops of the figure-of-eight. Such a protective barrier of light symbolizes that the space between the two people touches, but does not merge, while also protecting both against external influences.

Which technique of protection you choose is up to you – and of course there are many other possibilities from a range of traditions. Should you have the feeling, either before or after the massage, that undesirable energies have penetrated the protected space, you can remove them by mentally focussing your intention with the words, 'Return to your source, or be free!'*

* More on this topic can be found in Michael Gienger's *Purifying Crystals*, Earthdancer a Findhorn Press Imprint, 2008.

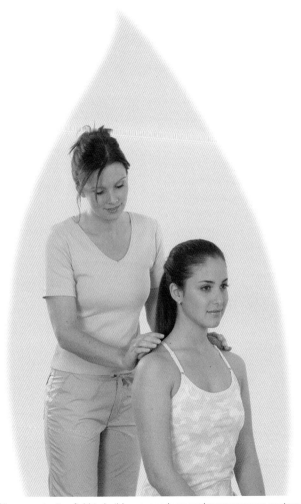

Allow a protective field to build up around you and your massage partner.

First Steps

(Please see note of caution on the following page.)

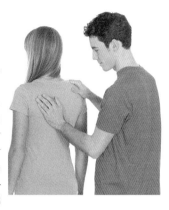

Now you can begin Joya® massage! For your first massage, begin with the shoulders and back. Take a moment to adopt an attentive and focussed attitude. Then, with your intuition as your guide, use your prepared Joya® roller to massage with stroking movements the muscles of the neck and shoulders, and anywhere you feel sufficient 'muscle mass', Maybe try out a few circling and kneading movements too. Do not hesitate to ask the recipient how it feels. No doubt you will quickly receive positive feedback as tension is often lodged in these areas. So, just vigorously knead the muscles, and also use outward stroking movements.

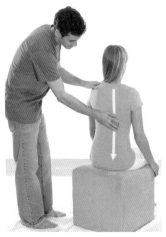

Next, carry on with the back. Stroke along the long back muscles a few times, to the left and right of the spine, from the neck down to the pelvic rim and upward again. As a rule, this feels really good and you will receive a positive response.

Please note: When massaging with crystal spheres, strong point-like forces can build up! Therefore never use the Joya® massage roller on the spine, neither on the neck nor back! Always move along the muscles to the right and left of the spine. The protuberances along the spine are very sensitive.

Generally speaking, you should always be extremely careful with bony areas and especially with joints, and only roll over them at 'zero pressure', or, if in doubt, don't touch them at all. Remain in the field of the muscles with your massage. They are usually very grateful for the attention!

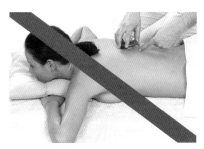

Never work directly on the spine!

Now you can expand to include other massage movements too; in addition to the stroking you have been doing, work through the muscles with circling, kneading, pummelling and rubbing movements. These are movements adapted from classic massage, and increase in intensity in the aforementioned order.

Always begin each new area with stroking movements, and then continue with circling, kneading, pummelling and rubbing movements. In between, always insert stroking movements so as to allow tension to flow away.

These five basic movements are explained again in detail on page 22, but, for the moment, we will remain briefly with your first Joya® back massage:

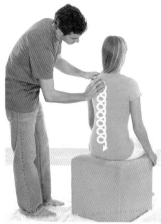

Circling

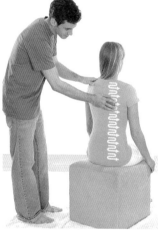

Pummelling

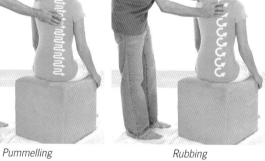

Kneading

Rubbing

After the long back muscles have been extensively worked on, you can carry on with the rest of the back. For example, use the roller to move a few times along the inner and lower edge of the shoulder blades and back again. That too, as a rule, is very pleasant.

Follow with the areas between the ribs, which should be stroked gently from the inside to the outside. Please proceed gently, as the ribs are very sensitive. The muscles between the ribs will be very grateful for the stroking.

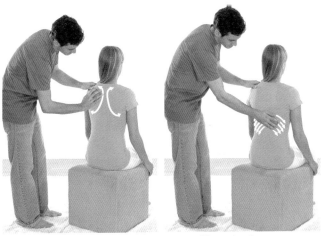

Massaging around the shoulder blades

Massaging the areas between the ribs

Next, massage the soft area between the rib cage and the pelvis, using different movements, but always with very little pressure   the kidneys, which are situated at the lower edge of the ribs, are also very sensitive.

However, the muscles that sit right at the upper edge of the pelvis can be massaged a little more vigorously. It feels good and is generally a great relief.

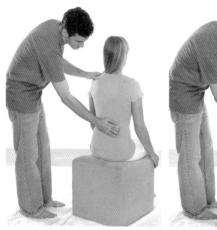

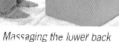

Massaging the lower back

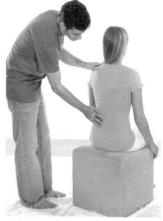

*Massaging the upper edge
of the pelvis*

Provided there is no sense that you might be invading the recipient's personal space, do not forget the large muscles in the buttocks. A number of muscles are situated there, all of which will be very thankful if something happens to them other than being sat on!

After that, you can essentially follow your own intuition. Simply massage with flowing, dynamic movements the areas where you intuitively feel your massage partner will benefit. Remain in the flow over the entire back, upwards and downwards. This kind of flowing 'rollering' is the speciality of the Joya® massage roller.

At the end, carry out a few gentle stroking movements on the neck and the shoulders again, as well as all over the back, and your first Joya® back massage is complete!

That was quite simple, wasn't it? Do ask your massage partner how it was. If you were sensitive and gentle, you are guaranteed to receive a positive response.

But beware of the insatiable ones, who immediately want more! Let's not rush things. And anyway, now would be a good opportunity to change roles so that you too can experience the pleasures of a Joya® massage! ☺

The Correct Hand Posture

After your initial experience with Joya® massage, you can begin to refine your skills a little, including the way you hold your Joya® roller. During the first massage, one is usually still intent on 'holding on' to the massage roller and therefore holds it too tightly. This, in turn, however, reduces sensitivity to the body being massaged. So, don't worry, just try laying your flat hand loosely over the massage roller as shown here:

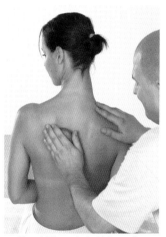

The right way to hold the roller:
loosely and relaxed!

If you lay your hand flatly and loosely over the roller, the fairly large area of contact alone will ensure that it remains securely in your hand! You will not need to hold on to it tightly, but will be able to use your fingers and the palm of your hand to make contact with the body in a relaxed manner. Thus your hand is able to feel, sense, perceive and direct the massage. This is the great advantage of Joya® massage: it is not your hands that have to do the work (the massaging is actually carried out by the roller and crystal sphere), and so you are able to use them totally as instruments of perception!

It is really worth comparing the difference: take the Joya® roller firmly in your hand, hold it with your fingers and then massage your lower arm or your thigh with it. How does that feel?

Then, place your hand loosely over the whole roller so that your fingers, palm and – depending on the movement – the edge of your hand all make contact with the part of the body being massaged. Then, once again, massage your lower arm or your thigh. Now how does that feel?

You can feel the difference, right? So, there you have it, you just learned the correct way of using the Joya® roller! Now we can proceed with refining the massage movements a little.

The Basic Technique of Joya® Massage

Thanks to the free mobility of the crystal sphere, as well as to the shifting of weight with the hand-piece, several very different movements are possible with Joya® massage. They have been named with reference to classic massage techniques.

Stroking: The roller is moved with little pressure, using shorter or longer stroking movements across the body. The stroking movements do not have to be straight all of the time and can include broader or tighter arcs. When stroking, we follow the lines and structures of the body with flowing movements. The stroking leads to a loosening and warming of all areas of the body, and can be carried out with a single roller or two in tandem. Excess energies and tensions are gently stroked out of the body.

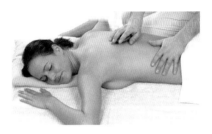

Circling: The roller is moved, with minimal pressure, in tighter or broader circling movements across the body so that loop-like movements are created. Tighter, faster circling movements have a stimulating effect; broader, slower movements have a calming and balancing effect. Circling also has a loosening, warming effect. As with the stroking movements, circling can be carried out with just one roller, or two in tandem.

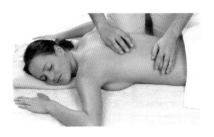

Kneading: Straight or circling movements are carried out while employing pressure rhythmically. The pressure exerted by the palm of the hand is a little stronger than when stroking and circling. The rhythm of pressing and letting go creates the kneading movement, which penetrates deeply into the tissue and muscle. Kneading with two rollers becomes particularly intense if bands of muscle are worked on from both sides at once. Kneading movements loosen tension and stimulate blood circulation.

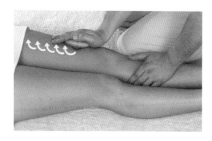

Pummelling: Deeper tissue layers or bands of muscle are worked on through back and forth shifting movements with a roller, or through parallel counter movements with two rollers. The pressure on the roller is noticeably stronger, compared with stroking and circling, in order to penetrate the deeper layers. Pummelling movements work on deeper levels, dissolving strong tensions and stimulating blood circulation.

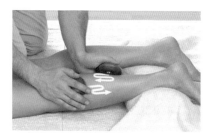

Rubbing: Rubbing consists of small, tight circling movements with firm pressure. Through using this movement almost 'on the spot', knots and swellings can be dissolved, and shortened tendons all around the joints can be worked on (the latter are often painful, so care should be taken!). Rubbing movements are for achieving great effect on deeper levels, and should therefore only be employed if the area in question has already been loosened and warmed up through other massage movements.

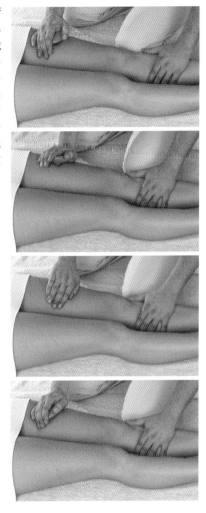

In order to ensure relaxation and avoid 'defensive' tension, each new area should be opened up first with stroking and circling, before kneading and pummelling. Please only use rubbing movements when the area has first been well massaged and warmed up. Smoothing outwards with stroking movements should also be interspersed again and again, in between other movements, so that energy released during kneading, pummelling and rubbing can flow away. This makes the relaxation process more effective.

First try out these five basic movements on yourself (while sitting, try them on your arms and thighs) and then with a massage partner. It is good to get to know all five movements, both by using them as well as receiving them. This will help you develop a sense of how each feels, and you will automatically learn to use the movements the right way – what feels good is 'right'!

All of these massage movements can be carried out both with a single roller or with two massage rollers in tandem. A massage with two rollers offers more possibilities and is often experienced as even more pleasant. Since it is often the case that only one roller is available, we have described all the massages in this book as using a single roller. Whenever you are using just one roller, please be sure to always keep your other hand in contact with the body of your massage partner. This just feels so much better for the person being treated!

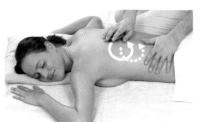
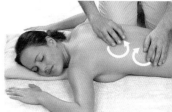

Massaging with one roller　　　　*Massaging with two rollers*

Full Body Massage

So, now you have reached the point where you can use the five basic movements to carry out a full body massage. Of course, you don't necessarily need to massage all the areas of the body mentioned in the following section, and you may shorten the massage if you wish. However, it would be good to try out all parts of the full massage, bit by bit, so that you can learn all aspects of it.

The total body massage begins, as before, with the neck, the shoulders and the back, and this time it is best done with your massage partner lying down. Pay attention to where and how each massage movement is used.

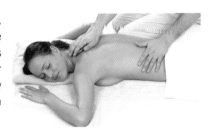

After the back, move on to the legs and feet. Begin with long stroking movements over the entire length of both legs down to the heels, or even to the soles of the feet. Afterwards you can massage the thighs, the calves, and, if desired, the soles of the feet, with circling, kneading, pummelling and rubbing movements from the top downwards. In between, repeat the outward smoothing (stroking movements) again and again.

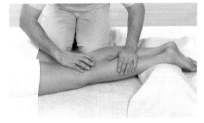

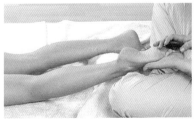

When carrying out a leg massage, please take note of the fact that the sides of the thighs are often more sensitive than the backs of the thighs, and also that the band of tendons below the twin muscles of the calves is much more sensitive than the muscle above. Likewise, you should also be very careful to decrease the applied pressure when moving across the hip joints, knee joints, and around the ankles.

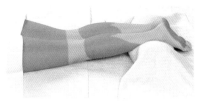

Pressure during leg massage:
red = more pressure, blue = medium
pressure, green= light pressure

After massaging the backs of the legs, you may ask your massage partner to turn over and lie on his or her back. As you are already massaging the legs, it is simplest to carry on. Begin at the front again with long, outward stroking movements from the top downwards and, similarly to massaging the back of the legs, follow with the other massage movements. But massage from the feet via the calves and the knee, rising up to the thighs.

When massaging the front of the legs, very carefully move around the outside of the kneecap with the roller.

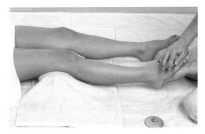

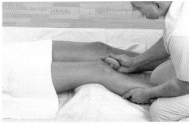

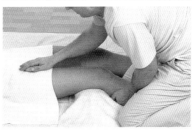

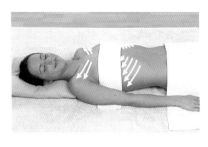

After the legs, move on to the chest and the stomach. For a woman, naturally only the chest above the breasts and the areas between the ribs on each side should be massaged, first with stroking movements and then possibly with gentle rubbing movements from the inside outwards. The often-neglected areas between the ribs on the side of the chest will be very grateful for a massage, as will the upper back area.

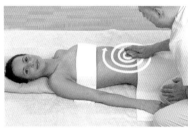

The abdominal area can be massaged with broad, sweeping, clockwise movements, stroking, circling and gently rubbing. You will be following the course of the large intestine, which rises on the right side of the body (seen from your perspective as the masseur as the *left* side of the body), then diagonally across the upper part of the abdomen, where it then descends again on the left side of the body (so on the *right,* from your point of view!).

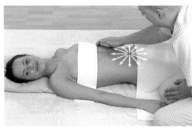

At the end of the abdominal massage you may carry out 'sun ray' stroking movements from the navel outwards. This is very pleasant and really does let the 'sun rise in the belly'.*

Now follow on with massaging the arms and hands in a similar way to the legs, being careful to handle the elbows and wrist joints very gently. Also massage between the bones of the hand on the back of the hand, very similarly to the areas between the ribs, and also gently pull the fingers with smoothing out movements. The palms of the hands are also very grateful for all variations of massage movements – a special treat you might like to save for the end of the arm and hand massage!

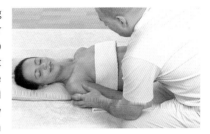

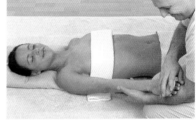

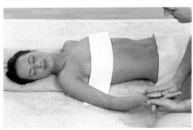

* This element of massage is derived from 'Crystal Balance' by Monika Grundmann. See also her book, *Crystal Balance*, Earthdancer a Findhorn Press Imprint, 2008.

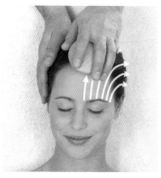

We finish the total body massage with the head and face. First stroke the forehead and the top of the skull on the left side, using parallel movements from the eyebrows outward towards the top. As you begin to approach the temple with these movements, start drawing the movement in an arc around the ear. Afterwards, circle around the ear a few times, and then massage the right side in the same way.

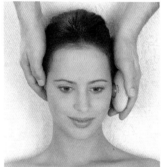

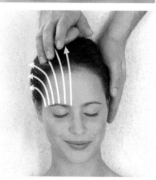

On the right side, proceed with the temple, the jaw muscles (this is where a lot of tension sits) and the cheek with circling movements. Back and forth stroking movements also feel very pleasurable underneath the cheekbone.

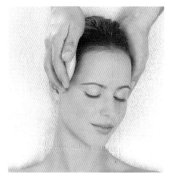

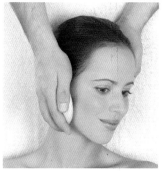

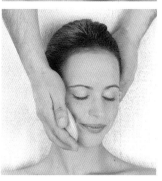

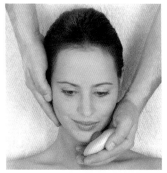

Stroke back and forth a few times across the lower jaw from one jaw joint to the other; also do this a few times under the chin, at the edge of the lower jaw, and very gently circle three times around the mouth.

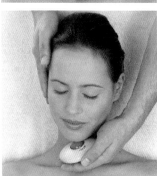

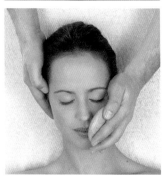

Change over to the left cheek so that stroking movements across the cheek, the cheekbone, the jaw muscles and the left temple follow one another.

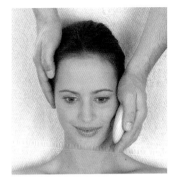

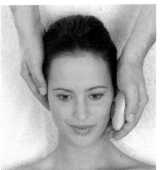

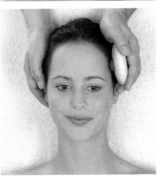

Starting at the left temple, circle around the eyes three times in a figure of eight movement: top edge of the right eye (underneath the eyebrow) – lower edge of the right eye – cross over at the bridge of the nose – top edge of the left eye (underneath the eyebrow) – lower edge of the left eye – change across the bridge of the nose, etc. Carry out this figure of eight movement several times – please, very gently and carefully. The movement ends at a point above the bridge of the nose, between the eyebrows.

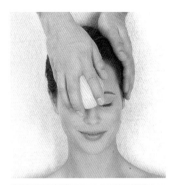

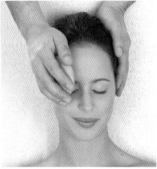

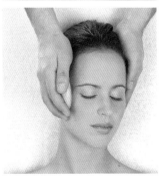

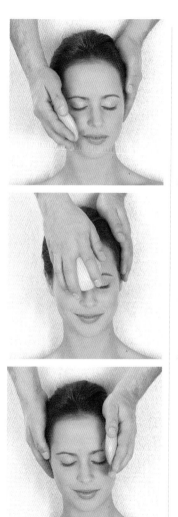
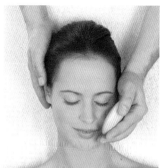
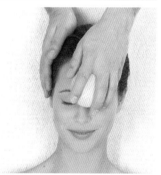

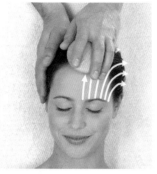

At the end, stroke the forehead and the top of the skull once again on both sides with parallel movements, as at the beginning of the head massage.

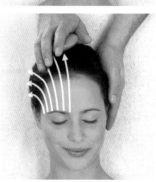

The full body massage is now finished. Allow your massage partner to rest for a little while afterwards, and take time yourself to enjoy the fact that you have just finished your first full body massage! And, isn't it true – anyone can give a massage!?

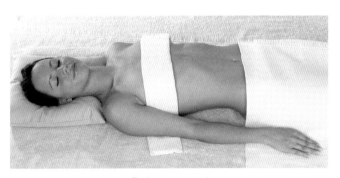

Post-massage rest

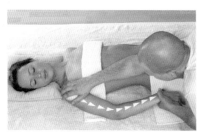

Rhythmic Flow

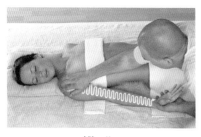

Vibrating

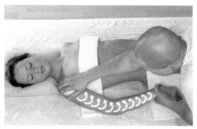

Rhythmic Arcs

Possibilities and Variations

Over time, the more massage you do the more familiar you will become with the five basic movements. You will learn quite naturally to adapt the movements according to the area of the body and the goal of the application, changing the pressure exerted, and changing the rhythm. From simple stroking you will move on to a rhythmic flow or even a vibration. From equal circles will flow a sequence of rhythmic arcs, and so on. When you have become familiar with the basic movements, every so often try out some 'modulations' on yourself; gradually you will be able to create your own repertoire of massage movements and penetrate ever deeper into the art of Joya® massage.

Along with the development of your skills, the repertoire of possibilities for applying Joya® massage will increase too. But before we turn to these possibilities and their practical applications, I would like to emphasize a very important point; there are definite 'contra-indicators', or situations when *not* to use Joya® massage. In massage, we must always remain aware of the boundaries as well as the possibilities.

When *Not* to Use Joya® Massage

Even though you may have had some successful experiences alleviating this or that minor complaint with Joya® massage, it is important to be aware that Joya® massage cannot replace medically necessary treatments and therapies! If physical or mental suffering is present, discuss with the treating physicians, naturopaths and therapists whether Joya® massage is appropriate. You need also be aware that massages might alter the effects of medications. For example, people with diabetes who have to take insulin should frequently check their blood sugar levels on the day of the massage, and the following day, in order to avoid any potential problems with low sugar levels. Also, before employing massage oils containing essential oils check for possible allergic reactions.

You should, generally speaking, refrain from carrying out a Joya® massage in the following cases:

- Raised temperature and infectious illnesses (including influenza and severe colds).
- Skin diseases over larger areas (especially eruptions on the feet or severe cases of Athlete's Foot).
- After a heart attack or a stroke. (Massage constitutes a heightened risk during the first 3-6 months.)
- Cancer patients (especially if they are receiving radiation or chemotherapy).
- People with pacemakers.
- Injuries, burns and recent operations.

- Undiagnosed or severe pain.
- Severe varicose veins, phlebitis, or bruising of the leg or foot. (There is a danger of blood clots being released and leading to embolisms.)
- Repetitive illnesses, such as rheumatism or multiple sclerosis.
- Lymphatic oedemas (also oedemas of the heart).
- Tendency towards attacks of cramp (also epilepsy).
- High-risk pregnancies – for lay people carrying out massages, one is generally advised to be extremely careful.

In principle, if you experience doubt about whether a massage would be appropriate, or whether you are the right person to give the massage, you should leave well alone! Even if the person begs. You would not be doing yourself or the other person any favours. In any of the above-mentioned situations, or if there are other vague or unclear symptoms, it is advisable to turn to people with expert knowledge.

When Joya® Massage is Perfect

Within a framework of the above guidelines and limits, there are still many areas of application where Joya® massage can help. Specific areas of application can be found in the next chapter.

A few general areas of application for Joya® massage:
- For general relaxation.
- To loosen muscle tension.
- To reduce stress and promote good sleep.
- To strengthen sight and hearing through relaxation.
- To alleviate tension headaches.
- To stabilize circulation, balance blood pressure.
- To improve blood circulation.
- To enhance supply of nutrients to and elimination from the tissues.
- For detoxification and elimination.
- For upright, well-balanced posture.

- To strengthen the spinal discs and the kneecaps.
- To calm and balance the nerves.
- For free, flexible joints.
- For general wellbeing.

This little volume is especially aimed at introducing how the Joya® massage roller can be employed for one's own preventative healthcare, for relaxation, wellbeing, and for the alleviation of minor complaints. However, please do not try to treat illnesses or more severe complaints on your own with the Joya® roller. Obtain expert advice in such cases.

Of course, we, the authors, would be very happy if physicians, therapists and alternative practitioners sought to allow patients to be actively involved in their healing process through the help of Joya® massage (but still under expert observation). Would it not be an optimal situation for patients to help themselves? This is why we would like to appeal to all those involved in medical or alternative treatments to please indicate your willingness to become involved out of your own initiative, and ask if you might employ the use of the Joya® massage roller.

But now let us now turn once again to the possibilities offered by the Joya® massage roller for improving your own health and wellbeing.

Joya® Massage

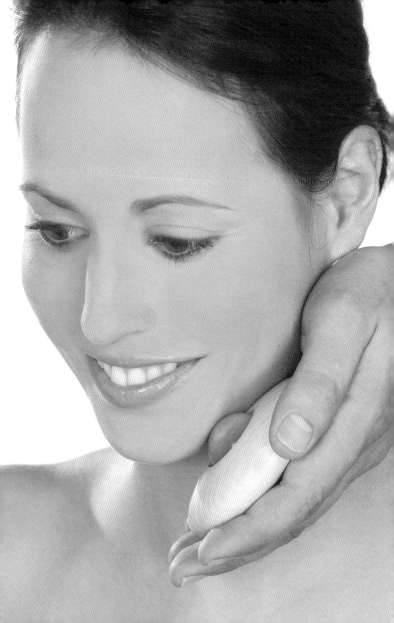

Joya® Massage

Joya® massage presents many possibilities for helping ourselves with the various physical problems that arise in everyday life (or for seeking help from a friend or relative). A number of these possibilities will be introduced in the following sections.

Muscle Tension and Complaints

Tense muscles? Muscular aches? Lack of energy? For these, Joya® massage can be a wonderfully effective solution. For muscle tension the best crystals to use are Amethyst, Dolomite, Magnesite, Serpentine, or Black Tourmaline (Schorl).

For a muscle hangover (after excessive activity), Dolomite, Landscape Jasper, Magnesite, Moss Agate, Nephrite and Serpentine are especially helpful.

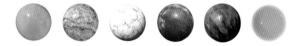

The Joya® massage roller can also be used as a preventive against muscle tension, or for building up muscles. The best crystals for these applications are Hematite, Red Jasper, Obsidian, Rose Quartz, or Stromatolite.

Do not only massage the muscle or area of muscles in question with the Joya® massage roller, also and always include:

- muscles located close by, or attached muscles (in the limbs);
- surrounding muscles (in the head, body and back);
- opposite muscles (on the right/left side of the body).

By doing so you will achieve holistic balance, which will have a deeper and more sustained effect.

Massage the muscles with alternating massage movements and always in the sequence: stroking – circling – kneading – pummelling – rubbing, as you learned in the back massage sequence (page 18 ff) and from the basic movements (page 22 ff).

Please take note of this sequence of massage movements, while remembering to repeatedly insert 'smoothing out' (stroking) movements in between. Details on this can be found in the section called 'The Basic Technique of Joya® Massage'.

Massage can be done anywhere – in lying, sitting or standing positions – depending on the area of the body and the situation. A few minutes of massage will often yield clear results. If the areas in question are easily accessible, the massage can also be carried out on oneself.

Tension Headaches

Do you get a headache after driving? After working at your computer? After reading in bad light? Tension headaches can occur around the eyes, but also rise up from the neck, the back, or even from the legs and feet (too much standing, or ill-fitting shoes, etc). Here too, Joya® massages are an excellent help! The best crystals spheres to apply are Amethyst, Aventurine, Nephrite, Rose Quartz, Serpentine, or Black Tourmaline (Schorl).

The best way, of course, is to receive this massage from someone else so that you can relax as much as possible. However, if this is not possible, you can massage yourself by simply doing the following:

Begin the massage while sitting, by massaging with 'smoothing out' movements from the forehead over the head, neck, shoulders and arms to the hands. Massage each side of the body with the opposite arm.

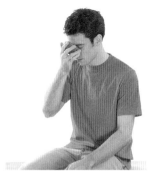

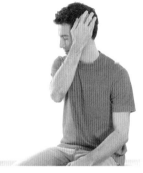

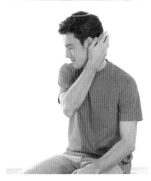

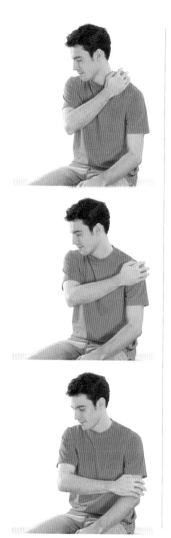

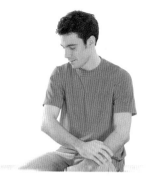

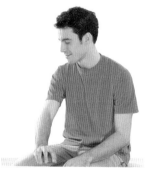

Next, if you can, lie down and massage the area around the eyes (forehead, temples, cheekbones), first with very gentle circling movements, then with stroking movements radiating from the eye outwards. If it is not convenient to lie down, do the same while sitting up.

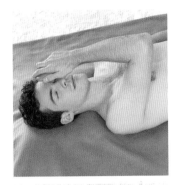

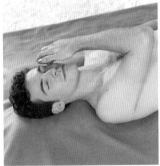

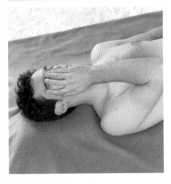

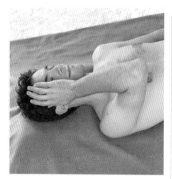

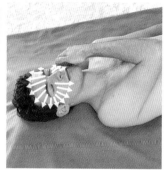

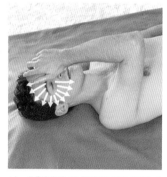

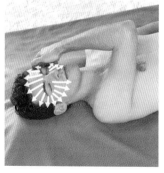

Now move around the eyes several times with a figure-of-eight movement – lower edge of the right eye – change over the bridge of the nose – upper edge of the left eye (underneath the eyebrow) – lower edge of the left eye – change over the bridge of the nose – upper edge of the right eye (under the eyebrow) – lower edge of the right eye, etc. Carry out this figure-of-eight movement several times, but please, very gently and carefully. The movement will end at the 'Third Eye', the point above the bridge of the nose between the eyebrows.

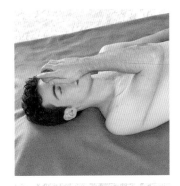

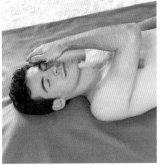

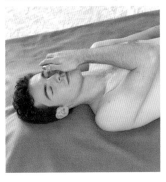

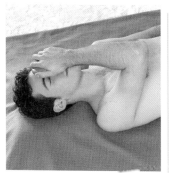 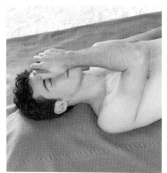

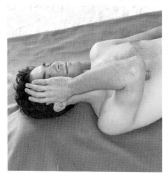

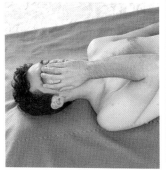

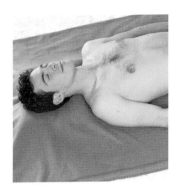

Remain lying down quietly for a few minutes, or sitting. Usually you will be able to observe how the tension headache gradually subsides.

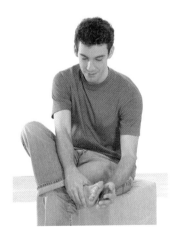

Please note: There are many different types of headaches. In the case of headaches based on metabolic problems, migraine, or other causes, this massage may not be effective or helpful. On no account should the treatment be continued if the headache becomes more severe. Also, for balance, it is advisable to massage the soles of the feet as well, so that any potential energy accumulation from the head area is drawn down to the feet. In the case of repeated headaches, visit a physician or alternative therapist and have the cause diagnosed!

Back and Spinal Disc Problems

Be sure the causes of the back complaint are diagnosed and treated therapeutically. A lack of expert treatment may lead to damage, but a therapy at the right time may prevent anything worse. Joya® massage may be helpful for alleviating symptoms and accelerating healing when used in conjunction with other therapeutic treatments. Certainly, regular massages will have a stabilizing effect and will enhance the healing process. Speak about this to the physician, naturopath or therapist who is treating the complaint.

Important: When carrying out a back massage, never massage on the spine itself! Only massage the long muscles to the right and left of the spine, and with great care and attention!

For back complaints due to tension, the following crystals are eminently suitable: Amethyst, Dolomite, Magnesite, Rose Quartz, or Serpentine.

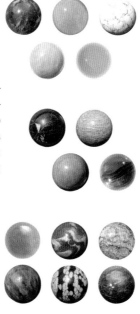

If a trapped nerve is involved, Black Tourmaline (Schorl) is the first choice of crystal, but Amazonite and Aventurine are also possibilities. In the case of complaints involving the spinal discs, Onyx Marble, a calc-sinter consisting of 80% Aragonite and 20% Calcite, is the absolute ultimate!

In cases of back complaints that go hand-in-hand with feelings of great exhaustion, Hematite, Red Jasper, Landscape Jasper, Nephrite, Obsidian and Sodalite can all be considered.

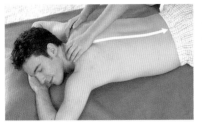

Carry out an extensive massage with the basic movements in the following sequence: stroking – circling – kneading – rubbing, as described on page 22 ff.

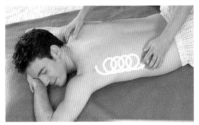

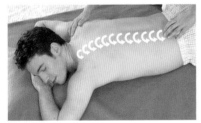

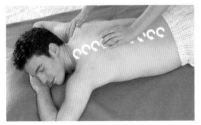

Back massage
(stroking, circling, kneading, rubbing)

However, carry out the final smoothing/stroking movements across the buttocks and the legs, right down to the feet, toes, and even beyond them.

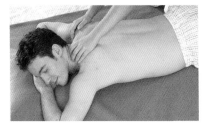

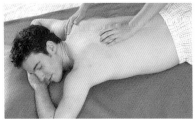

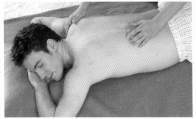

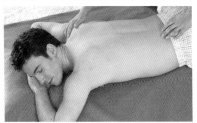

The final smoothing out movements

Joint Complaints

Our joints are generally given very little attention – that is, until they hurt! Yet they are of the greatest importance for our flexibility, and for the flow of energy within the body. The metabolism, vessels, muscles, sinews, nerves and energy channels (meridians) interplay closely at the joints. Blocked joints can therefore result in negative side effects in almost all parts of the body.

Joya® massage in the areas of the joints should be very, very gentle. The goal is an energetic stimulation of the metabolism to build up the substance of the joints, eliminate deposits, release energetic blocks, harmonize the nerves, and relax the muscles and sinews. For all of this, no pressure is required – on the contrary, too much pressure will have an over-stimulating effect and would thus be damaging! It should also be noted that one should never massage directly on top of the bony and cartilaginous parts of the joints, but always around them.

The most suitable crystals for massaging the areas of the joints are Amazonite, Aventurine, Dolomite, Landscape Jasper, Onyx Marble, Snow Quartz and Black Tourmaline (Schorl). Onyx Marble is the No. 1 best crystal for complaints of the kneecap!

First circulate around the joint in question with calm movements and minimal pressure, and then stroke away from the joint outwards with short stroking movements.

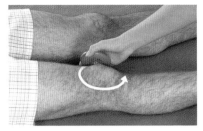

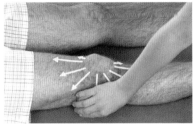

Massage the area around the joint with very slow, gentle, circular movements, flowing gradually to *very gentle* rubbing. When rubbing commences, the movements will become smaller and a little firmer. However, they should never come anywhere even close to the pain threshold!

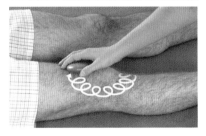

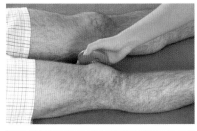

Next, with free movements, massage the area around the joint just as it feels right and good for the person being massaged. Follow the contours of the body in arcs, loops and curves – just as it comes naturally.

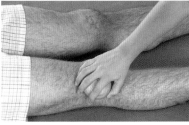

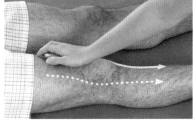

To finish, stroke out the entire area around the joint while 'elegantly' moving around the actual joint. Smoothing out should be done from the top downwards, or in the case of the limbs, always in the direction of the hands/fingertips or feet/toes.

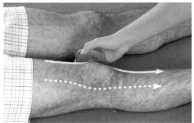

Tip: The Joya® massage will work best if you combine the associated elements of the full body massage with the joint treatment. So in the case of elbow joint complaints, for example, it is best to massage the entire arm from the shoulder to the fingers. In the case of a knee problem, massage the whole leg from the hip down to the toes. And, if at all possible, also treat the same joint (or area) on the other side of the body. Where the symptoms are more severe, it is actually better to massage the 'good side' of the body first.

General Tension and Stress

Tense? Stressed? Allow yourself a Joya® massage with a crystal sphere made of Amethyst, Magnesite, Rose Quartz, Serpentine, or Black Tourmaline (Schorl).

You can carry out this massage either with another person or as a self-massage, and we will present both possibilities here.

Self-massage: Using smoothing out movements, massage from the forehead over the head, neck, shoulders and arms, down to the hands.

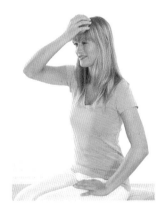

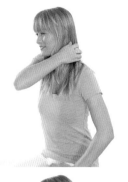

Next, massage the legs in the same way from the hips down to the tips of the toes. At the end, allow yourself the pleasure of an extensive massage of the soles of your feet, using circling, kneading and rubbing movements. By this point, at the very latest, all tension and stress will have evaporated.

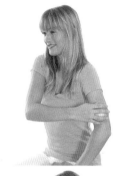

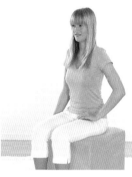

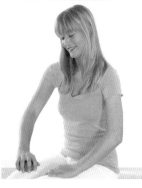

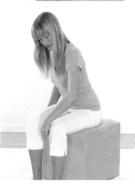

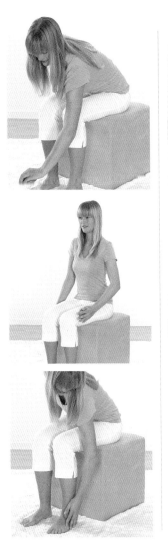
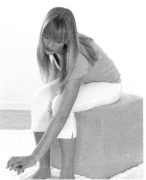
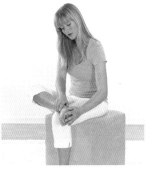

If you wish to conduct the massage more extensively, or deepen it, massage the areas of the body mentioned just as you did in the full body massage – partial areas of the head (but not the face), shoulders, neck, and legs (fronts only). For the arms, use only the smoothing out movement. You will need to adapt the massage movements so that they are conducted from the top downwards, and you are able to carry them out in a relaxed manner.

Massage with a partner: Use smoothing out movements to massage from the forehead across the head, neck, shoulders, back, legs (backs and outer edges) to the feet. Finish the massage with an extensive treatment of the soles of the feet with circling, kneading and rubbing movements.

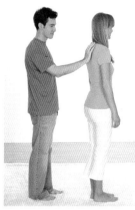

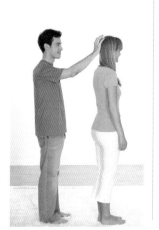

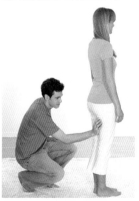

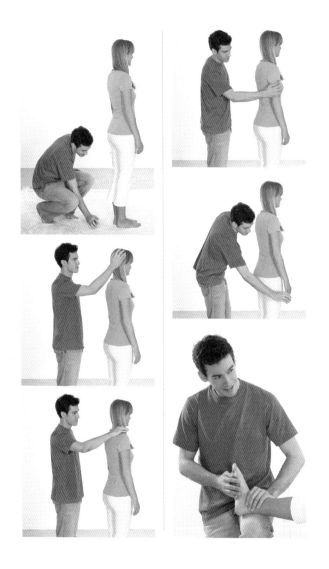

Here, too, you may conduct the massage in a more extensive or deepening manner by massaging the parts of the body mentioned as you did in the full body massage – partial areas of the head (but not the face), shoulders and neck, back as well as legs (backs). Adapt the massage movements in such a way that they are directed from the top downward, and, right at the end, smooth out (stroke) along the entire length of the body.

Sleep Problems

Do you find it difficult to switch off and go to sleep? Do those pesky thoughts keep going round and round in your head? Are you dead tired, but sleep will just not come? Or do you wake up feeling as though you have not slept deeply? Through deep relaxation, as can be achieved with a Joya® massage, you will go to sleep more easily and sleep more deeply. Many sleep problems can be completely eliminated if you also pay attention to your rhythms of sleep and, if necessary, make changes to the place where you sleep so as to remove the possibility of further disturbances.*

Crystal spheres suitable for treatment of sleep issues are Agate, Aventurine, Dolomite, Magnesite, Rose Quartz, Serpentine and Black Tourmaline (Schorl). However, Rose Quartz stimulates sensuality and so might in fact prevent one from sleeping...

* Michael Gienger, *The Healing Crystal Fist Aid Manual*, Earthdancer a Findhorn Press Imprint, 2006.

Self-massage: First massage your legs while seated. You may combine different movements such as stroking, circling, kneading and pummelling, according to what feels good to you. However, always massage from the top downward and then stroke out extensively from the top downward. This will encourage tension to flow out.

Next, massage the soles of your feet (stroking, circling, and kneading), using very calm movements and very gentle pressure. (Strong pressure is stimulating.) You are massaging the polar opposite of the head, which will therefore calm your thoughts.

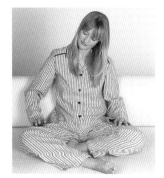

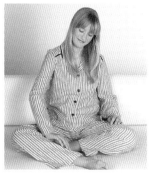

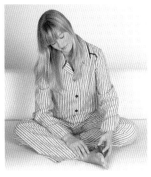

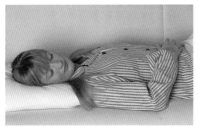

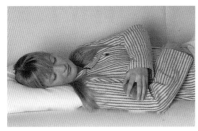

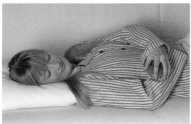

Now lie down in bed, turn out the light, and then very calmly begin massaging your abdomen. Use stroking and circling movements, with pressure that feels most comfortable for you. After that, massage your arms from the shoulder joint towards the hands. Use mainly smoothing out, and maybe a few clockwise circling movements.

You may find that during the arm massage the roller will almost drop out of your hand. As an alternative, you can use gentle circular movements on the temples and end the massage with smoothing out movements on the forehead. The smoothing out movements always follow the line of the eyebrows upward across the forehead and the head.

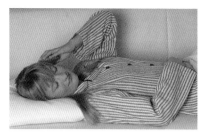

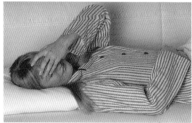

When you have finished, lay the roller aside and remain lying down without turning the light on again. Sleep will definitely come faster than usual.

Possibly try out different types of crystal on different nights. The best success rate has been achieved with Aventurine, followed by Black Tourmaline (Schorl), which is especially helpful if the disturbing influences of radiation and electro-magnetic pollution might be playing a part.

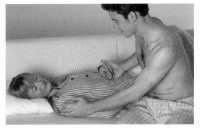

Massage with a Partner: For a partner massage we will change the sequence. (For the self-massage, the massage of the legs was carried out first for practical reasons.) Here we start with the arms, then the abdomen, then the legs. Right at the end, if desired, the temples, the forehead and the head are massaged. The recipient should ideally already be lying in bed with the lights dimmed.

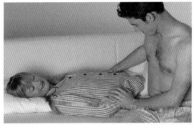

Begin with the right arm, massaging from the shoulder joint to the hand. Use mainly smoothing out and gently circling movements. Spend some time on the palm of the hand with stroking, circling and kneading movements. At the end, stroke out the fingers with a 'corkscrew' movement, and finally, stroke out the entire arm and the hand. Now do the same for the left arm.

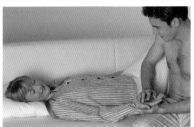

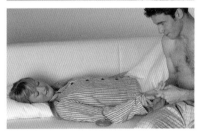

Next, move in a flowing manner to the abdomen and massage initially with large circulating movements with a flat hand (clockwise!). Then take the Joya® massage roller and massage using small, very calm, circular movements, following a route that runs along the course of the large intestine (a broad clockwise circle) and then around the entire abdomen, spiralling inwards and then outwards again until the abdomen has once again been circled along the course of the large intestine. All these movements must be clockwise, including both the small circling movements with the roller, as well as the spiral courses, moving inwards and outwards!

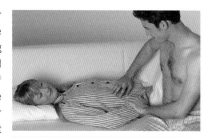

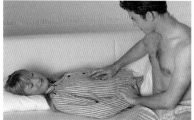

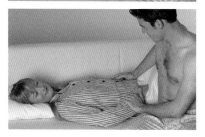

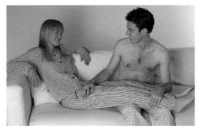

Usually it will suffice to massage the abdomen once using this inward and outward spiral course. If your massage partner clearly displays an expression of well-being, you may carry on and perform this abdominal massage up to three times.

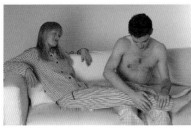

Proceed now with a flowing transition to the right leg, and massage it from the top downward, from the hip joint to the foot. You may combine various movements such as stroking, circling, kneading and pummelling, according to your own judgement, but smoothing out beyond the foot should be the dominant element throughout! The smoothing out process will cause a lot of tension to flow away. Afterwards, massage the left leg in the same way.

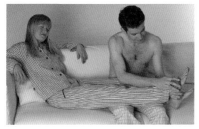

Next, using very calm movements (stroking, circling and kneading), massage the soles of the feet with very gentle pressure (stronger pressure will have a stimulating effect). Massaging the feet, as they are the polar opposite of the head, will calm thoughts. This can be supported by making the massage movements more and more gentle and fine until they can hardly be felt. Fortunately, the crystal sphere in the Joya® massage roller is almost never perceived as 'tickly'.

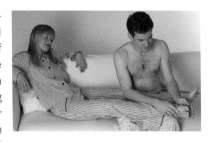

If the person you are massaging is becoming visibly relaxed and sleepy while having their feet massaged, end the massage there. Otherwise you can very gently massage the temples (in circling movements) and then stroke out from the forehead across the head. The stroking movements should always run from the line of the eyebrows upward.

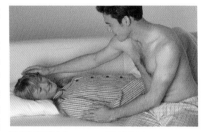

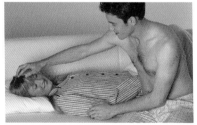

Tiredness

Do you often lack energy and feel tired, even if you have had enough sleep? Do you feel as if you are not up to meeting present stresses or imminent challenges? You can mobilize your energies with the following Joya® self-massage and drive away tiredness! This massage is a self-massage, as DIY is an essential element of it.

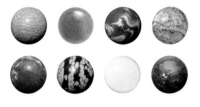

The best crystal spheres for this 'Hey, wake up!' massage are Amazonite, Hematite, Red Jasper, Landscape Jasper, Moss Agate, Obsidian, Snow Quartz, and Sodalite.

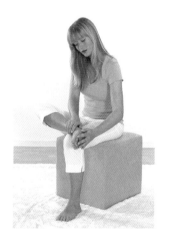

Start in a sitting position and perform a short, vigorous massage of the soles of the feet. Freely combine massage movements as you wish (stroking, circling, kneading, pummelling, rubbing). Keep all the movements brief and vigorous.

Next, massage first the calf of the left leg with fast up and down movements, and then repeat the same with the right leg. After that, shake out each leg vigorously.

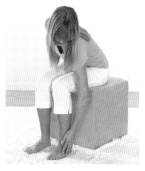

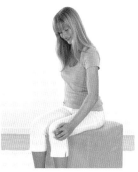

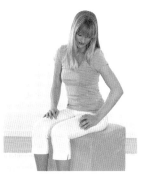

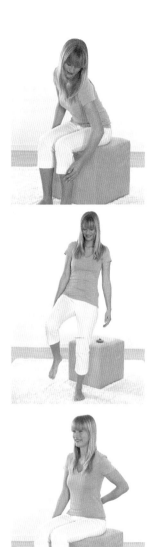

Then massage the buttocks, and especially the sacrum, with circling as well as upward and downward stroking movements. Adapt the pressure so that it feels pleasant to you, but keep the movements energetic!

After that, massage the abdomen with broad circular movements, which, seen from the front, proceed clockwise, and then stroke a few times up and down across the solar plexus and the sternum.

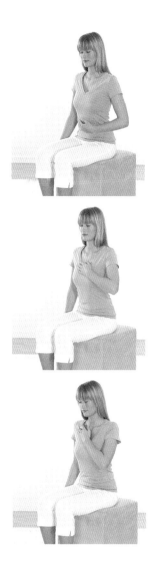

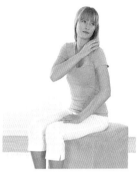

Proceed in a flowing manner to the left arm and massage it on all sides, again with fast up and down movements. Then do the same with the right arm.

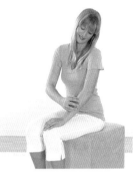

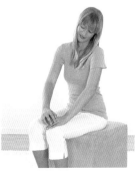

Then remove the crystal sphere from the Joya® massage roller and roll it between the palms of your hands and closed fingers. Put quite a bit of pressure on the sphere and make the movements fast.

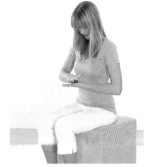

At the end, vigorously shake out both arms at the same time.

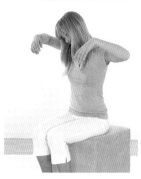

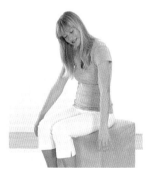

If you like, you may also shake out your entire body for twenty to thirty seconds. Your body will have been switched back to active mode and you'll find some pep has returned to your life!

Circulation Problems

You can use the Joya® massage roller with upward and downward movements to work on circulation problems. High blood pressure is alleviated if the downward movements are emphasized. Emphasizing the upward movements will stimulate the circulation and will thus raise low blood pressure.

If you are taking medication for circulation problems, please consider possible interactive effects and talk about this with the physician or naturopath who is treating you.

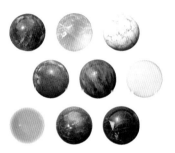

Suitable crystal spheres for a Joya® massage for treating high blood pressure are Amethyst, Clear Quartz, Magnesite, Moss Agate, Nephrite, Snow Quartz, Serpentine, Sodalite, and Black Tourmaline (Schorl).

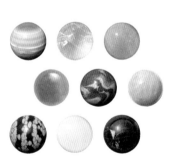

Suitable crystal spheres for a Joya® massage for treating low blood pressure are Agate, Clear Quartz, Dolomite, Hematite, Red Jasper, Rose Quartz, Obsidian, Snow Quartz, and Black Tourmaline (Schorl).

Clear Quartz, Snowy Quartz and Black Tourmaline (Schorl) are 'neutral', and will therefore help with high or low blood pressure depending on whether the massage is carried out with emphasis on upward or downward movements.

Joya® massage for high blood pressure and low blood pressure can, in principle, be carried out both as self-massage or with a partner. For treating high blood pressure the partner massage is ideal as it is more passive, while the more active self-massage better suits the treatment of low blood pressure. For this reason, the massages are described in this way. However, depending on the situation, they can also be carried out the other way around.

Massaging a Partner with High Blood Pressure: This massage is best carried out while the partner is standing up. Place the Joya® massage roller in the centre of the forehead (on the 'Third Eye'), or on the head, and pass it along the centre of the body across the top of the head and then down to the right of the spine in the neck and the back, over the right buttock and down the leg to the ground. There draw it back and away, as if you were drawing out and conducting away excess energy.

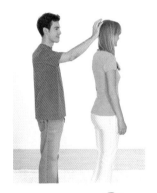

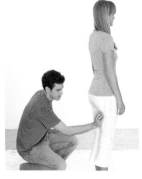

Attention: Be sure to move alongside the spine and never massage directly on it!

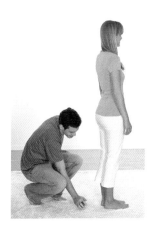

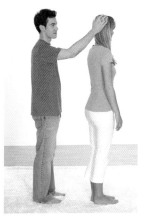

Now place the Joya® massage roller one centimetre to the right of the 'Third Eye' beside the eye brow, or once again on the head, and pass it parallel to the centre of the body across the top of the head and then down to the right of the spine in the neck and back, over the right buttock and down the leg to the ground. There, again, draw it back and away as if removing excess energy. This second course should be taken about one centimetre from the first course on the head and neck, and about two to three centimetres beside the first course on the back and the leg, depending on the dimensions of the person's body.

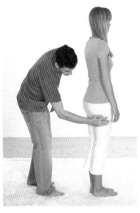

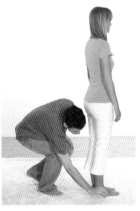

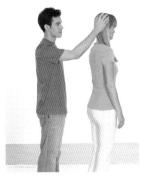

In this way, you will be prescribing one parallel course after another, next to the previous one. The final courses, which are carried out near the temples, or start on the temples and run right around the ear, will no longer pass over the back and down to the legs, but across the shoulders to the arms and the hands.

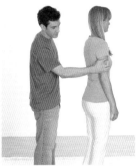

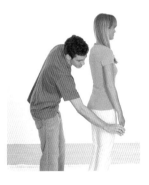

Then start again with the 'Third Eye', or on the head, but pass the Joya® massage roller to the left of the spine down to the ground. Further courses run parallel to the centre of the body on the left side.

The entire Joya® massage with all the parallel courses on the right and left sides of the body can be repeated up to three times and, in extreme cases, even more.

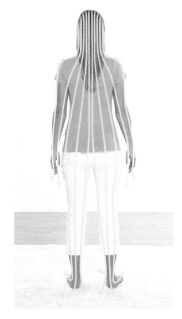

This smoothing out massage releases tension and energy blocks, which will also visibly lower the blood pressure. The most obvious results were achieved with Amethyst, Moss Agate, and Sodalite. Tests showed that in people with normal or low blood pressure, this massage can lead to dizziness and even the experience of blackness in front of the eyes through plummeting blood pressure. In such cases, the limbs should be vigorously massaged with fast upward movements, which will immediately normalize the circulation once again.

For the self-massage, pass the Joya® massage roller in parallel lines, always proceeding from the head, across the shoulders, arms and hands. Afterwards, massage your legs with vigorous downward movements and finally massage the head once again as described above. Self-massage is best carried out while sitting.

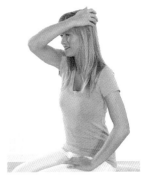

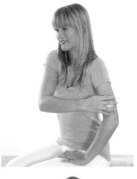

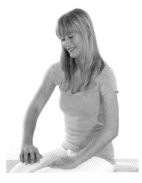

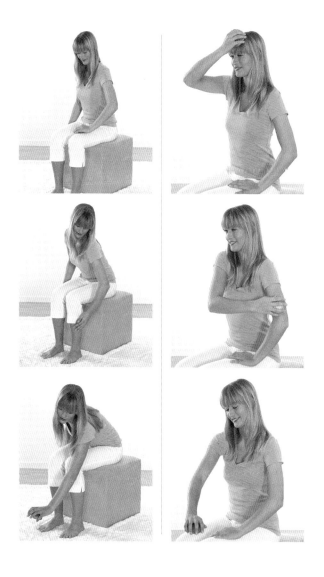

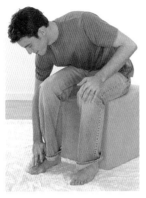

Self-massage for treating low blood pressure: While sitting, first massage the right leg, then the left leg, with vigorous movements from below upwards. Throughout, alternate stroking, circling and kneading movements according to how you feel. However, it is important that you carry out strong upward stroking movements again and again.

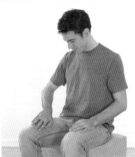

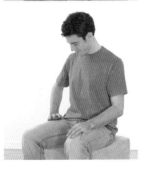

Then massage the sacrum with circling as well as with downward stroking movements. You will need to adapt the pressure so that it feels pleasant, but the method of carrying it out should remain energetic!

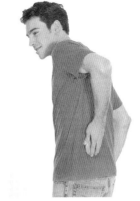

Next, massage the abdomen in large circular movements, which run clockwise when seen from the front.

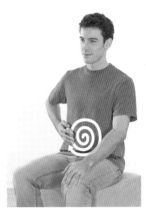

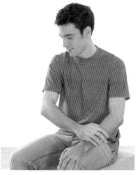

Then stroke a few times across the solar plexus (the centre of body above the navel) and the sternum with up and down movements, and then proceed in flowing movements to the right arm. Massage the arm on all sides with similar up and down movements. Emphasize the upward movements, which may lead across the shoulders to the neck. Massage the left arm in the same way.

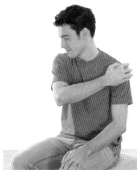

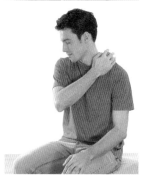

To end, use very gentle circular movements to massage your temples, then hold the Joya® massage roller with its crystal sphere on the point between the eyebrows (the 'Third Eye').

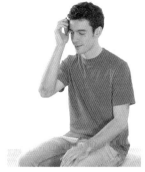

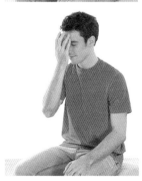

If at any point during the massage you have the impression that your blood pressure is rising (feeling of warmth, perception of rising energy, or similar), stop massaging at that point. If you feel that the pressure or the rising energy is getting too much for you, bring balance by massaging your limbs with rapid downward strokes.

Circulation Problems in the Limbs

Do your arms or legs often 'go to sleep'? Do you suffer from chronic cold hands and feet? Regular Joya® massages may be an effective and consistent help. They can be carried out as self-massage or with a partner. For simplicity's sake, the massage will be described here as a self-massage.

The best crystal spheres for treating circulatory problems in the limbs are Dolomite, Hematite, Red Jasper, Landscape Jasper, Obsidian, Rose Quartz, and Stromatolite.

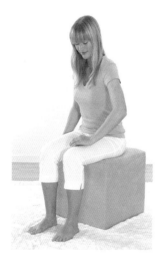

Start with massaging your legs from the hip joints to the feet, using gentle and rather slow up and down stroking movements with medium pressure. After that, massage the soles of your feet with vigorous pressure, starting with circular movements, then kneading and then rubbing. First massage the left, then the right foot – possibly alternating several times until both are perceptibly warmed and 'softened'.

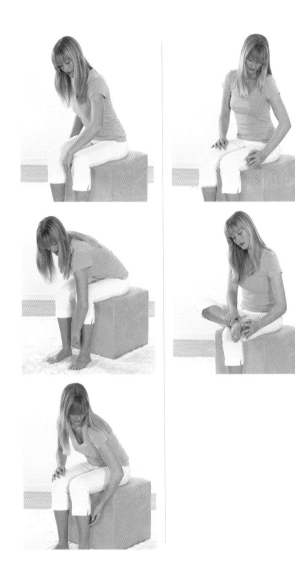

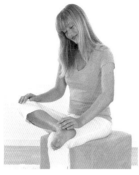

Then focus on the areas of the inner and outer ankle of both legs, massaging with free movements in any way that feels comfortable.

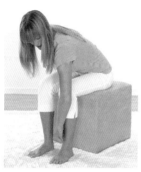

Then continue the massage up to the knee, first on the left leg, then on the right leg, with slow circling, kneading and rubbing movements and medium pressure. The important thing is that the leg is being warmed up.

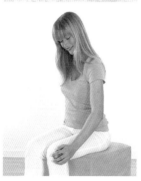

Massage the entire knee area of both legs with free movements, in a way that feels good for you. You may also stretch or bend the knee several times, to make it 'permeable' for energy and warmth.

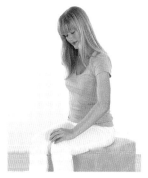

Massage the thighs up to the hip joint, once again with slow circling, kneading and rubbing movements, with medium to firm pressure (depending on how you feel).

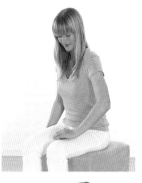

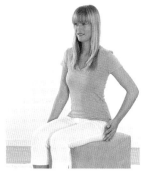

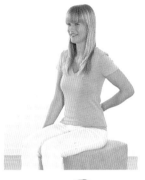

After that, massage your sacrum with circling movements. Adapt the pressure so that it is comfortable for you, and carry out the movements gently and calmly.

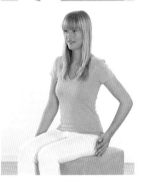

From the sacrum, move the Joya® massage roller across the left buttock and down the side of the left leg, and then follow with several calm, downward, stroking movements on all sides of the leg.

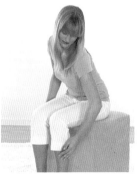

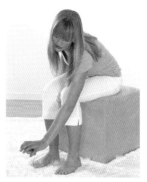

Then massage the right leg in the same way.

Move on to the arms. Begin by massaging your arms from the shoulder joint down to the hands with gentle and rather slow up and down stroking movements and medium pressure.

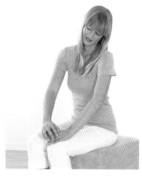

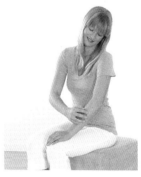

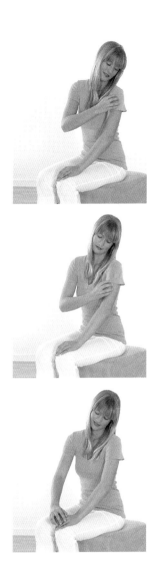

After that, massage the palms of your hands with firm pressure, initially with circling movements, then with kneading and rubbing. First massage the left hand, then the right hand – possibly even alternating several times, until both are perceptibly warmed up and 'softer'. Then shake your hands out vigorously.

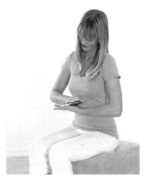

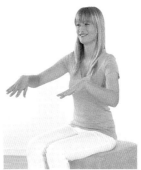

Massage the entire wrist with free movements, as feels good to you.

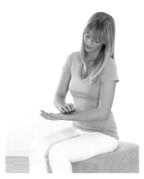

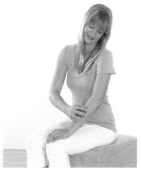

Continue the massage up to the shoulder joint, first on the left arm and then on the right, using slow, circling, kneading and rubbing movements and medium pressure.

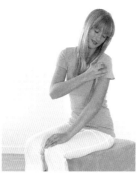

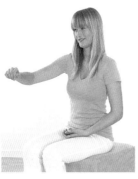

You can also stretch and bend the elbow joint in between, or move it several times, in order to make it 'permeable' for energy and warmth.

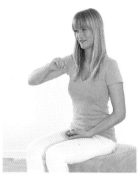

At the end of the arm massage, circle around the shoulder joint several times.

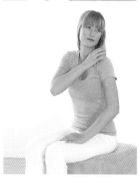

If you like, at this point you may also vigorously shake out your entire arms.

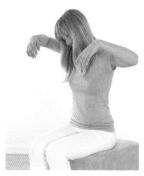

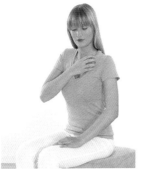

Continue the movement around the shoulder joint, flowing under the collarbone to the sternum, stroking the latter up and down several times.

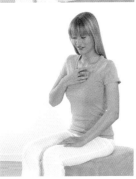

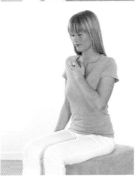

From the sternum continue the movement under the collarbone to the left shoulder joint, circle around it several times and return to the sternum.

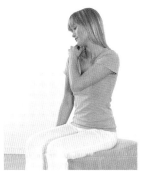

Massage the areas of both shoulder joints in this way, alternating several times and returning back to the sternum again and again in between and stroking up and down.

Finally, pass the Joya® massage roller from the sternum downward to just above the navel and then begin circling around the navel very gently and calmly in a clockwise direction (seen from the front).

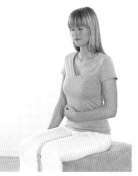

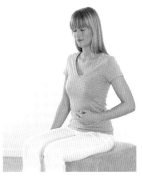

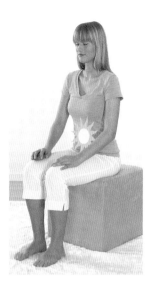

Allow the circling movement to become gradually larger and larger, until the entire area of the tummy between the ribs and the pelvis has been massaged. Then gently lift off the roller.

Remain sitting quietly for a while and observe how the warmth streams out from your tummy into your limbs. Imagine a Sun in your tummy ... the rays filling your limbs and warming your hands and feet. Enjoy this feeling as long as you like!

This massage strengthens the energy regulation system of our organism (called the 'triple warmer' in traditional Chinese medicine) and improves blood circulation. If desired, the leg and arm massages may also be carried out separately. However, always end with an abdominal massage and the image of the 'sun in your tummy'.

Detox and Elimination

Behind many physical complaints – skin problems, frequent infections (colds, etc.), allergies, to name but a few – are often hidden toxins deposited in the connective tissues.* Here, too, Joya® massage can promote the detoxification and elimination processes, and effectively support other therapeutic measures such as diets, fasting cures or medical treatments.

Crystals recommended for detoxification and elimination are Amazonite, Aventurine, Clear Quartz, Landscape Jasper, Moss Agate, Nephrite, Sodalite, Stromatolite, and Black Tourmaline (Schorl).

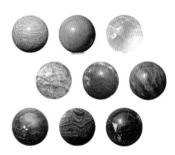

As detoxification and elimination are both total body processes, we recommend the Joya® full body massage described in the previous chapter – with the crystal spheres mentioned above. If a full body massage is too time-consuming or not possible for other reasons, we recommend a massage of the front of the body (chest, tummy and legs), or at least a massage of the organ zones on the abdomen.**

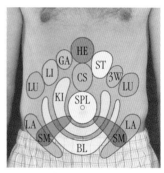

The organ zones

* see Michael Gienger, *The Healing Crystal First Aid Manual*, Earthdancer a Findhorn Press Imprint, 2006
** The 'organ zones' are reflexology zones of the functioning circles of the body according to Chinese medicine.

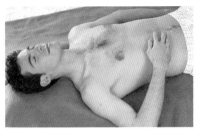

The ideal time for a massage of this kind is the late afternoon or evening so that the body can continue with the detoxification and elimination processes overnight.

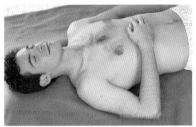

Massage of the organ zones can also be carried out as a self-massage! Once you have become more familiar with the individual zones, you can even carry out the massage while lying down in the dark before going to sleep.

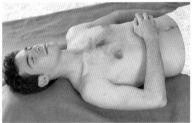

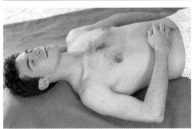

The organ zones are massaged clockwise in four 'circles', using circling and kneading movements.

Outer circle: Lung zone right (LU) – Liver zone (LI) – Gall bladder zone (GA) – Heart zone (HE) – Stomach zone (ST) – Triple Warmer zone (3W) – Lung zone left (LU) – Large Intestine zone left (LA) – Small Intestine zone left (SM) – Small Intestine zone right (SM) – Large Intestine zone right (LA).

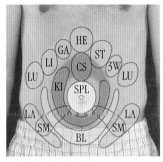

The four circles of the organ zones

Second circle (semi circle): Bladder zone (BL).

Third circle: Circulation-Sex zone (CS) – Kidney zone (KI).

Inner circle: Spleen zone (SPL).

Give attention to each zone until you feel the movement has become easier and freer, or until you sense a feeling of wellbeing emanating from the zone in question. If the massage of a particular zone feels very uncomfortable or unpleasant, move on and come back to it later for a second course of the 'four circles'. In this way, the mutual blocks in the different organ zones will be released.

Through a reflective harmonisation of the internal organs the entire metabolism will be balanced with this massage, which will ease considerably the detoxification and elimination processes. When there are indications of a blocked detoxification process (headaches, painful limbs, diarrhoea), this particular Joya® massage may provide some relief, as it boosts the elimination process and very gently supports the detoxification of the tissues.

Important: After a Joya® massage with detoxifying and eliminating crystal spheres such as Moss Agate or Nephrite, it is essential to drink lots of water! At the minimum, drink half a litre or a whole litre of water immediately after the massage, and two to three litres daily during the following few days. And 'water' here means 'water', not any other kinds of drinks.*

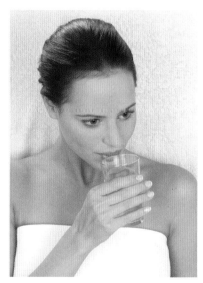

Drink good water!

* Michael Gienger/Joachim Goebel, *Gem Water*, Earthdancer a Findhorn Press Imprint, 2008

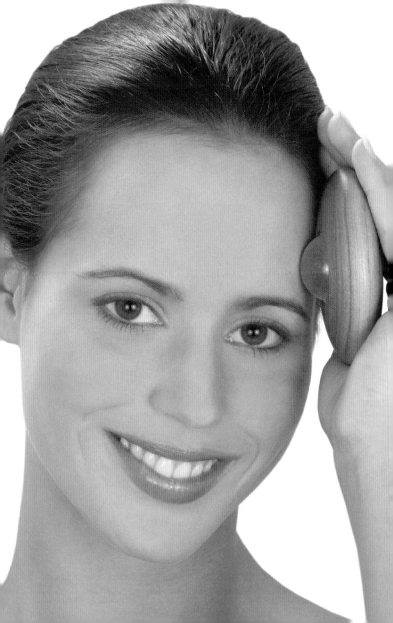

The Effects
of Various
Crystal Spheres

The Effects of Various Crystal Spheres

The following 'portraits' briefly summarize the effects that have been observed using different crystals in Joya® massage. Although an astonishing abundance of effects have been recorded, just a few years of observations are by no means enough to create a comprehensive 'portrait' of each crystal. Thus our descriptions do not claim to be complete. They also do not illustrate the entire spectrum of effectiveness of the crystals, more of which may have been observed in other crystal healing applications (laying on, wearing, gem water, etc.). Instead we will steer you towards the relevant resources, and focus instead on the results that relate mainly to Joya® massage.*

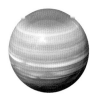 **Agate** firms up and strengthens the connective tissues and supports the functions of the skin. It improves the processes of supply, elimination and detoxification of the tissues, as well as digestion and elimination in general. In this way, Agate helps regulate the metabolism. As it is a crystal containing Chalcedony, it has a mildly stimulating influence on the lymphatic system. Agate can be applied for massage in all areas of the body. It is very popular for use on the arms as it creates a feeling of calm, reflective vigour. Agate is also well suited for massaging the tummy as it has a protective and gently stimulating effect on nearly all the internal organs. The feeling of protection and security provided by Agate also helps bring about calm and refreshing sleep.

* Michael Gienger, *Crystal Healing*, Cassell (Blandford), London, 1998
Michael Gienger, *The Healing Crystal First Aid Manual*, Earthdancer a Findhorn Press Imprint, 2006
Michael Gienger/Joachim Goebel, *Gem Water*, Earthdancer a Findhorn Press Imprint, 2008

Amazonite helps with the effects of tension and cramp, such as tennis elbow and carpal tunnel syndrome. Central issues for this crystal are: narrowing, stiffening, hardening of the muscles, chronic tension, and neuralgia that has arisen through excessive burdening, continuous irritation or mechanical demands. (Tourmaline is preferred for actual nerve injury.) Amazonite improves the flexibility of the joints, helps with complaints connected with the tendons and thus, thanks to its eliminating effect, also helps with rheumatic complaints. It helps with liver problems and chronic tiredness. ('Tiredness is the pain of the liver' says an old German saying.) It is used especially for massage of the neck, shoulders and arms, and sometimes also for the back or the tummy.

Amethyst alleviates pain. It is useful for conditions with symptoms that include strong, acute or chronic muscle tension, especially tension around the eyes, tension of the jaw muscles, tension headaches or back problems. It also brings visible relief to sprains, twists, pulled ligaments and muscles, and swellings. In massage, amethyst can be applied to all areas of the body. Amethyst also lowers blood pressure in cases of circulation problems. It helps with stress and the consequences of stress, has a liberating effect when used to massage the chest area, makes breathing easier and releases feelings of anxiety. In the tummy area it supports the activity of the large intestine and helps with diarrhoea. As it is a clearing, purifying crystal, Amethyst is also very suitable for the skin and for massaging the tummy.

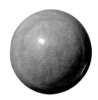

Aventurine alleviates general conditions of tension and cramp, especially chronic tension with side effects such as tennis elbow and carpel tunnel syndrome, among others. Aventurine can also be used for tension headaches or irritated nerves. It alleviates rheumatic complaints of the joints, purifies the connective tissues and the skin, and, as a liver-fortifying crystal, has a regulating effect on the metabolism. Aventurine has also been tried and tested in cases of headaches associated with metabolic problems, as well as those that arise from excessive exposure to the sun (sunburn and sunstroke). It is one of the best crystals for the entire body, and magically bestows a 'new face'. It can be used for neck and shoulder massage, as well as for the occasional back massage. Aventurine massages help clear the mind of bothersome thoughts, and thereby help with getting to sleep and sleeping through the night.

Clear Quartz is a neutral massage crystal that bestows clarity and energy. It is very useful in a diagnostic massage to help determine the condition of certain areas of the body, reflexology zones, and the causes of acute and chronic tension. Clear Quartz purifies the skin and firms up the connective tissues. Due to its neutrality, it is ideally suited for massage of the various organ zones of the tummy. Clear Quartz is often used in facial massage as a cooling crystal on the area around the eyes. It is also used for the gentle elimination, lymph mobilization and pain alleviation achievable through so-called 'drawing out through the nerves'. In addition, Clear Quartz has a regulating effect on the thyroid gland, can be used to release tension in the chest area, and can be applied to stimulate the circulation.

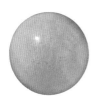

Dolomite alleviates muscular 'hangovers', cramp, and muscle tension. It is especially helpful whenever tension affects the internal organs. Dolomite is therefore often a favourite crystal for tummy and back massage when internal organ involvement is suspected or confirmed. The equilibrium of the elements Calcium and Magnesium in Dolomite make it an excellent regulator for the metabolism, the blood pressure and circulation in the tissues, and muscle tone. It can also be applied for problems in the joints (especially in the arms) and postural damage (incorrect posture, 'favouring'). Dolomite bestows a sense of satisfaction with oneself and the world, alleviates stress and thereby also improves sleep.

Hematite is applied for circulation problems, chronic tiredness and major exhaustion. It clearly lowers blood pressure if the massage is carried out vigorously; with more gentle massages, it strengthens the blood circulation in the tissues and the supply to the tissues. It improves muscle build-up and is therefore used specifically for massages of the limbs, but also for the back and the tummy. In the latter case, strengthening and functional activation of many internal organs can be observed, particularly the liver, kidneys and small intestine. In the area of the heart it sometimes has *too* strong an effect, so avoid the chest area. Also care and attention is advised if there is inflammation or infection.

Red **Jasper** is employed for circulatory problems. It is a little 'milder' than Hematite and has a muscle strengthening and blood pressure raising effect. It supports the blood circulation in the tissues and the supply of nutrients to them, and is often used for the massage of the limbs, as well as for the back and the tummy. Use it for an arm massage to bestow a feeling of strength and energy. It helps generally with tiredness and exhaustion, and has a warming and enlivening effect. In the case of tummy and back massages, Red Jasper activates the liver, the kidneys and the small intestines. According to Chinese medicine it activates the 'Triple Warmer'.

Landscape Jasper supports digestion and elimination (good for tummy massages!). It improves the supply to and elimination from the connective tissues, as well as, to a lesser extent, their detoxification and elimination processes. With long-term application, it strengthens the immune system and calms allergies. Landscape Jasper fortifies the limbs, keeps the joints flexible, and helps with stress, tiredness and exhaustion. It is popularly used for arm massage. As it stimulates the metabolism and the blood circulation in the tissues, it is useful for calming muscular hangovers.

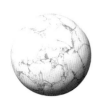

Magnesite alleviates pain, stress, and general conditions of tension and cramp. It helps with back problems, tension headaches, high blood pressure and migraines; and can be used in a targeted way for lack of magnesium (cramp in the calves!), muscular hangover, localized muscle tension, as well as the consequences of accidents (for example, sprains or pulled ligaments and muscles). Because it stimulates the metabolism, Magnesite supports the processes of supply, detoxification, elimination and purification of the tissues. It can be used almost anywhere on the body. It is especially well suited to the massage of organ zones on the tummy because it relaxes the internal organs, and even alleviates colic. The deep relaxation afforded by Magnesite also improves sleep.

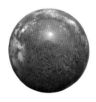

Moss Agate helps with chronic tension and burdened connective tissues, which are often indicated by water retention or skin problems. As a mineral from the Chalcedony family, it can generally be employed to improve the lymph flow, and thus supports the tissues in the processes of supply, detoxification, elimination, and drainage. Thus Moss Agate regulates the metabolism and the blood pressure, fortifies the immune system, and helps with infections, colds and ear complaints. Moss Agate also stimulates activity in various glands in the body, which is why it also lifts hormone-related tiredness. Moss Agate is popularly used to massage the limbs (lymph flow, muscle hangover, pain in the limbs), the head and chest area (colds, immune system, etc.), as well as the tummy (metabolism).

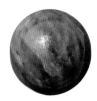

Nephrite improves blood circulation and water distribution in the head, and thus helps with tiredness, but also with serious illnesses such as tinnitus and migraine. It also encourages recuperation during difficult periods. Nephrite is excellently suited for treating the tummy. It strengthens the liver and the kidneys and thus has an eliminating, metabolism regulating, and blood pressure lowering effect. Nephrite stimulates the lymph flow, improves the supply to and the elimination from the tissues and thus has a purifying effect on the skin. It helps with muscular hangover, problems of the spinal discs, and chronic tension that affects the internal organs. It can also be used for tension headaches. In massage, Nephrite is used from head to toe!

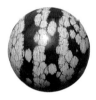

Obsidian can be applied for the consequences of accidents (for example, sprains and pulled ligaments or muscles) and for the alleviation of pain and shock. It is also extremely helpful after operations, and generally for blocked wound healing (in acute situations, however, only under medical supervision!). Obsidian helps with circulatory complaints, supports the blood circulation in the limbs (even in cases of hardening of arteries in the leg due to smoking), and helps with chronically cold hands and feet. It helps with lack of energy, tiredness, extreme weakness, and lack of drive; it strengthens and enlivens the muscles and is therefore used particularly for massage of the limbs, but also for the back and the tummy. The latter visibly leads to a stimulation of the organs of elimination – the kidneys, the bladder, and the intestines.

Onyx Marble can be applied for chronic tension and complaints of the spine. It strengthens the muscles and encourages their activities. With its high Aragonite content (80%), Onyx Marble also has a regenerating effect on the spinal discs and the kneecaps. For this reason, it is also one of the most important crystals for joint complaints (especially for shoulders, hips, elbows and knees), as well as damage due to incorrect posture and 'favouring'. Onyx Marble is used particularly for massaging the back and the limbs. During massage of the stomach and abdominal area, it stimulates the metabolism (especially the calcium metabolism) and alleviates digestive problems.

Rose Quartz harmonizes the heart rhythm, and stimulates a healthy heart to achieve balanced, vigorous activity. However, if heart problems are present, one should never treat the person without first consulting a physician or naturopath. Rose Quartz encourages warmth, sincerity and sensuality and is, therefore, unlike the generally held opinion, only sometimes, but not always, a soporific. It does, however, reduce stress, helps with the balance between activity and relaxation, and sensitizes one towards one's own mental and physical needs. This also makes it a very pleasant crystal for a tummy massage. Rose Quartz strengthens the muscles and renders them flexible, alleviates chronic tension, strengthens the circulation, and improves the tissues' blood circulation and supply of nutrients. This leads to healthy and rosy-hued skin. Rose Quartz has a particularly relaxing effect on the face, which leads to a beautiful and pleasant radiance. This relaxing effect may also encourage the alleviation of tension headaches.

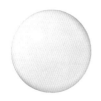

Snow Quartz is a very neutral, gently energizing crystal. It helps with tiredness and, during a massage of the chest, alleviates breathing blocks that have arisen through tension and stress. Snow Quartz has a calming effect on internal restlessness and alleviates pain (but only minor pain). Snow Quartz is very pleasant for spinal and joint problems (especially if the joints often feel cold and then easily become painful). It is also helpful for weakness and sensations of numbness in the limbs. It is favoured for massaging the arms and hands. Snow Quartz purifies and firms up the skin and can be employed for stimulating the lymphatic system and the circulation.

Serpentine (trade name 'China Jade') encourages detoxification and elimination, is particularly good for de-acidifying, and alleviates muscular hangover, pain, and states of tension and cramp. It can be used to target cramp due to lack of Magnesium (cramp in the calves!). It helps with tension in individual muscles, and also with tension headaches and back problems. Green Serpentine relaxes muscle tension, which has a further beneficial effect on the internal organs, and can also be applied directly for cramp and colic in internal organs (outstanding for tummy massage!). Using this crystal for massage can also rapidly bring relief from menstrual pain. Green Serpentine is applied in all areas of the body. It has a blood pressure lowering effect, bestows inner peace, brings balance to internal states of stress, and improves sleep.

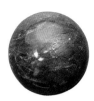

Sodalite regulates the water balance, thus encouraging the functioning of the lymph flow and the supply to the tissues, and the detoxification and elimination processes of the tissues. It has a cooling effect on both external and internal heat, lowers blood pressure and regulates perspiration. Sodalite is very good for the skin and can be used wherever there is too much or too little moisture. It strengthens the kidneys and thus also helps with feelings of tiredness, exhaustion and burn out. Sodalite has a gently relaxing effect and is also good for tired, burning eyes. It has a harmonizing effect during tummy massages, and is also a favourite for tired feet, and for leg massages in general.

Stromatolite is a wonderful crystal for tummy massage. It loosens tension and cramp, but also has an activating effect when lack of energy and slowed functioning of the internal organs is present. This makes it, among other things, an excellent helper for sluggish intestinal functioning. Stromatolite stimulates the entire digestion and elimination processes; it also balances the metabolism, improves the blood circulation, improves the supply to and elimination from the tissues, and gently stimulates detoxification and elimination. It is particularly effective for the firming up of connective tissues and for strengthening the muscles.

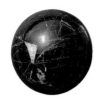

Black Tourmaline (Schorl) alleviates all kinds of states of tension and cramp, also tension headaches, breathing blocks, and urine retention. It also helps with constipation, nausea and other symptoms caused by stress, tension and chronic tension. Black Tourmaline can also be applied for postural damage, joint problems, sprains, pulled ligaments or muscles, etc., as well as for alleviating pain and reducing problems due to scarring. It is also helpful for tension that has lead to consequences such as tennis elbow, carpal tunnel syndrome, and much more. Also, Schorl can be applied if the nerves are affected as well, which means it can be used for neuralgia and sciatica. Black Tourmaline can also help with the effects of radiation from cell phones, transmission towers, computers, etc.; and in this context, too, it relieves tension and improves sleep. Depending on the manner in which it is applied, Schorl can also be used to regulate the circulation. It is a wonderful crystal for massage, but sadly only very rarely available as a Joya crystal sphere due to the fact that raw crystals suitable for polishing into a sphere shape are not readily available.

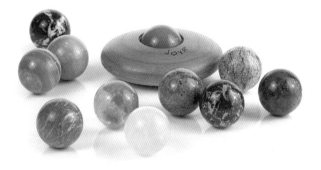

Final Tips and Information

Final Tips and Information

In order to expand the range of uses for Joya® massage rollers, special rollers have been developed in addition to the Joya® Classic featured in this book. These are the Joya® Professional, the Joya® Mini, the Joya® Massage Pen and the Joya® Massage Glove.

The Joya® Professional is very similar to the Joya® Classic, both in its shape and use. The only real difference is that the hand-piece is made out of a mineral composite (minerals and acrylic) that can be thoroughly cleansed and disinfected. This is particularly important for its therapeutic use in natural healing or in professional massage, but is also advantageous for Joya® massages carried out with oil (see page 130).

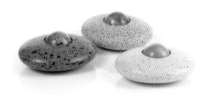

Joya® Professional

The Joya® Mini consists of a small, cylindrical hand-piece with an integrated movable crystal sphere. You can use the same crystal spheres as for the Joya® Classic. The Joya® Mini is, however, more flexible for use in certain areas of the body (face, neck, joints, etc.). The Joya® Mini also has a lid, making it ideal for travel! This small roller is also available in a mineral composite, and is called the Joya® Mini Professional.

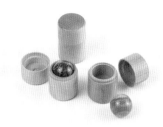

Joya® Mini

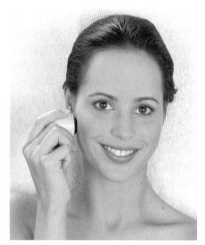

Joya® Mini in action

The Joya® Massage Pen was originally developed for facial massage. Crystal spheres with a diameter of 15mm are more suitable for massaging the 'nooks and crannies' of the face, for example the areas around the eyes. The pen shape makes it easier to perform massage movements in areas where the Joya® Classic would have restricted access and movement possibilities. This functionality has led to the Joya® Massage Pen being used extensively in areas other than the face as well.

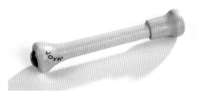

The Joya® Massage Pen

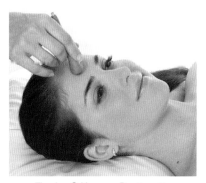

The Joya® Massage Pen in action

The Joya® Massage Glove consists of a washable fabric with a crystal sphere inserted in a socket at the centre of the palm of the hand. The crystal sphere is not held in place with a Teflon ring this time, rather it moves freely in the socket. Body contact with the crystal sphere is enhanced, and there is free movement in all directions. Using the Joya® Massage Glove you can massage both manually and with a crystal sphere. The possibilities for such a Joya® massage are truly boundless.

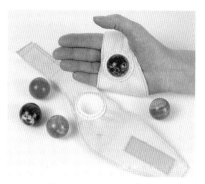

The Joya® Massage Glove

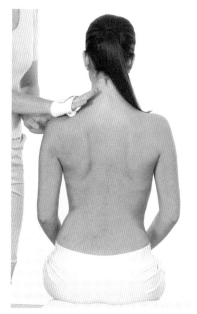

The Joya® Massage Glove in action

High quality massage oils, especially if they are warmed up, generally make a massage even more relaxing, and also encourage elimination from the skin. This only applies to pure plant-based, high quality oils – the best being from controlled, organically grown sources. Oils based on petrochemicals are pure poison; they clog the pores of the skin and then actually lead to blockages. The best experiences we have had in terms of using oils in Joya® massage – also from the angle of allergy avoidance – were with sesame oil for the body and almond oil for the face.

Oils in which crystals have lain are a particular pleasure. If a high quality oil and a well-cleansed (purified) crystal are placed together in a warm spot for a long period of time, the oil will absorb information from the crystal and thus develop its effects. If you choose an appropriate crystal sphere for a Joya® massage, the theme of the crystal and the oil will be enhanced and the Joya® massage will have its own special note.

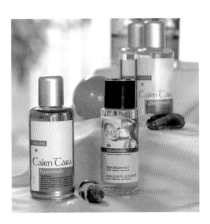

We recommend the gem oils developed by Monika Grundmann, which bring together the effects of crystals and the properties of essential oils.

(Available in the specialist trade or through Farfalla Essentials*.) We also recommend the Cairn Tara Crystal Gem Oils with herbal extracts developed by Franca Bauer (Maienfelser Naturkosmetik). These gem oils are also obtainable in the specialist trade.

Joya® Massage with Warmed Crystals

The greatest pleasure and sense of wellbeing and the deepest reaching effects are achieved with Joya® massages with warmed crystal spheres! The crystal spheres are either pre-warmed in a bath of water above a tea-light burner, in warm massage oil, or on a bed of sand with a warming dish. A Joya® massage with warmed crystals is a real delight, from the very first touch!

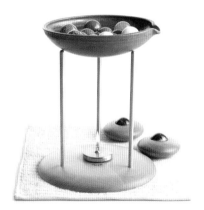

Please Note!

When warming the crystal spheres in massage oil over a burner or on a bed of sand, very high temperatures can occur. The oil and the crystals could lead to burns if they are not handled in an expert and knowledgeable way. Please do not exceed the optimal temperature of approximately 35° C!

* See www.naturaleurope.com and www.crystal-balance.com

The Joya® Warming Pillow

The Joya® Warming Pillow is made from organic cotton with organic grain filling. It can be heated by placing it on a radiator (or in the oven) (50° C max.), and will remain warm for a long time. Joya® Warming Pillows allow you to pre-warm the massage roller and crystal spheres, and/or to gradually warm the area of the body to be massaged. There is a special pocket sewn into the pouch to house the roller.

Just imagine having two warm pillows placed upon your neck and shoulders, and then receiving a massage with a warm roller and spheres – heaven!

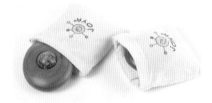

Joya® Warming Pillows

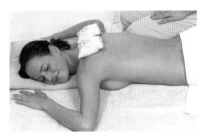

*Joya® massage of the neck
with two Joya® Warming Pillows*

Cleaning Your Joya® Massage Roller

When it comes time to clean your massage roller, extract the crystal sphere using the suction cap (gem remover). The hand-piece can then be cleaned, if necessary, with warm water and an organic washing up liquid,* but should be rapidly and thoroughly dried afterwards so that the wood does not swell. We highly recommend using the washing lotion developed by Monika Grundmann (the founder of 'Crystal Balance'), which is available from a number of sellers.

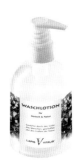

If you wish to use massage oil in your 'Joya® massages we recommend using the Joya® Professional which is made of a mineral composite and therefore much easier to clean. The material is not harmed by washing up liquids and is heat resistant, and can therefore be washed with hot water to remove traces of oil, and can be disinfected.

The crystal spheres themselves can be cleaned with warm soapy water or the above-mentioned washing lotion, but under no circumstances should aggressive, acid-containing cleansing agents be used! Otherwise, crystals such as Dolomite, Hematite, Magnesite and Onyx Marble will develop a rough surface and are then no longer suitable for the roller. If desired, the spheres can also be disinfected with alcohol.

After cleaning, the crystal spheres should be cleansed of any 'information' or energies they may have absorbed. Simply hold them under running water for about a minute, dry them, and then lay them for a few hours on a piece of Amethyst druse or use a complete Amethyst druse. The 'crystal lawn' of Amethysts possesses a high-frequency radiation that is able to remove 'foreign information' in other crystals.

* See also Monika Grundmann's *Crystal Balance*, Earthdancer a Findhorn Press Imprint, 2008; also www.crystal-balance.com

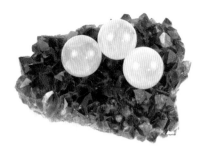

Energetic cleansing on Amethyst

Alternatively, the crystal spheres may be placed in a small glass dish, which, in turn, is bedded in a larger dish of salt. Salt also has an energetically cleansing effect; however, the spheres should only be laid on salt in this way for a maximum of two to four hours, otherwise the salt may have a 'leaching' and weakening effect *

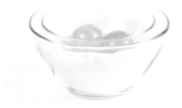

Energetic cleansing with salt

After this cleansing procedure, the Joya® massage roller can be re-assembled and used for the next massage.

** More on the subject of cleansing can be found in Michael Gienger's *Purifying Crystals*, Earthdancer a Findhorn Press Imprint, 2008.

Appendix

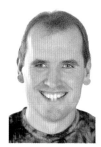

Michael Gienger worked as a shiatsu masseur before entering the field of crystal healing in the late 1980s. Massage with crystals has thus been part of his work for more than twenty years. His research into crystal healing, which created the foundations of 'Analytical Crystal Healing', has earned Michael international acclaim. As an author he has published some twenty works, a number of which have become standard reference works in this field and have been translated into eleven languages so far. In addition to his activities as an author, and publisher of Edition Cairn Elen with the German publisher, Neue Erde, Michael Gienger also gives lectures and seminars on crystal healing and related fields. You can find out more about Michael Gienger and his projects at: www.michael-gienger.de, www.fairtrademinerals.de, www.cairn-elen.net, www.steinheilkunde.de

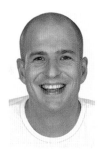

Ulrich Metz was born with an immense creative streak. Over the last fifteen years, before developing the Joya® massage method, Ulrich worked as a sculptor, using and combining materials in a way that reflects a highly developed feel for sensory opposites. Glass and metal, wood and stone, bone and metal, bronze and marble – there are very few materials available to sculptors that Ulrich has *not* explored and combined.

Ulrich Metz lived in South Africa from 1995 to 1996 and there deepened his knowledge and sensitivity for the connections between humans and natural materials. It was also there that he first encountered the healing powers of crystals.

Though some years later, these direct and personal experiences became the impulse behind the Joya® massage roller. Since then, Ulrich has further developed the Joya® principle into other products, which have expanded the possibilities for massage still further.

You can find out more about Ulrich Metz and Joya® at: www.joya.eu

Thanks

Our thanks go especially to those people who, through constructive criticism and input, have contributed towards the further development of Joya® massage since the publication of our first book. We would also like to thank all our colleagues and employees working with the Joya® principles, who patiently cared for and assured the quality of each of the Joya® products. We thank all those masseurs, women and men, who have taken Joya® out into the world, and are sharing the pleasure, joy and sense of wellbeing that can be derived from using the rollers. Special thanks also go to those who have supported and cooperated with the content of this book – Ewald Kliegel, Ellen Bendin and Sabine Schneider-Kuehnle. Heartfelt thanks go to Ines Blersch for her wonderful photographs, as well as to Jens Ville for assistance in the photo studio. We also thank our models, Carmen Weiers, Janka Vogt, Raphael Crespo, Ludmila Fraia and Marion Schnatterbeck for their commitment and cooperation, and to Stefan Fischer for finding Carmen and Marion. Our final thanks go to Fred Hageneder for the graphics and layout, and to our publisher, Andreas Lentz, who patiently carried the project forward, although once again it took three months longer than originally planned...☺

Picture Credits

Ines Blersch (www.inesblersch.de): all photo illustrations except for the following:
Lapis Vitalis® (www.lapisvitalis.de): page 133

Literature

Crystal Massage

M. Grundmann, *Crystal Balance*, Earthdancer a Findhorn Press Imprint, 2008

N. Kircher, *Gemstone Reflexology*, Inner Traditions, Rochester, 2006

E. Kliegel, *Crystal Wands*, Earthdancer a Findhorn Press Imprint, 2009

Crystal Healing

M. Gienger, *The Healing Crystal First Aid Manual*, Earthdancer a Findhorn Press Imprint, 2006

M. Gienger, *Crystal Healing*, Blandford, London, 1998

M. Gienger, *Healing Crystals*, Earthdancer a Findhorn Press Imprint, 2005

M. Gienger, *Purifying Crystals*, Earthdancer a Findhorn Press Imprint, 2008

M. Gienger, J. Goebel, *Gem Water*, Earthdancer a Findhorn Press Imprint, 2008

Joya® Massage Rollers

Joya® Massage Rollers, Joya® Massage Pens and accompanying crystal spheres can be found in the mineral specialist trade, as well as in the specialist trade for wellness, cosmetics and health products. Up-to-date information on this: www.joya.eu

Crystal Massage Oils

Crystal massage oils by Monika Grundmann (Farfalla Essentials) and Cairn Tara Crystal Oils with herbal extracts (Maienfelser Naturkosmetik) can be found in the specialist trade for wellness, cosmetics, and health products.

Seminars and Training

Joya® Massage

Information on Joya® Massage Rollers and other products, as well as on seminars and training for Joya® Massage:

Joya® International

Ulrich Metz, Gerberstrasse 9, 64625 Bensheim, Germany
Tel: +49 +49 (0) 700 569 29 675
info@joya.eu, www.joya.eu

Akademie Lapis Vitalis®

Im Osterholz 1, 71636 Ludwigsburg, Germany
Tel: +49 +49 (0) 7141 44 12 60, Fax: +49 (0) 7141 44 12 66
seminare@lapisvitalis.de, www.lapisvitalis.de

Huldersun Akademie

Klaus & Ute Schmidt-Hüser

Dorfstrasse 10, 37574 Einbeck-Hullersen, Germany

Tel: +49 (0) 5561 71 815, Fax: +49 (0) 5561 31 39 153

info@huldersun.de, www.huldersun.de

Farfalla Essentials AG

Florastrasse 18, CH-8610 Uster; Switzerland

info@farfalla.ch, www.farfalla.ch

Crystal Massage and Crystal Healing

Consultations on crystal application, seminars, basic and advanced training sessions for crystal healing, crystal massage and related fields.

Cairn Elen Lebensschule Tübingen

Annette Jakobi, Bachstrasse 87, 72810 Gomaringen, Germany

Tel: +49 (0) 7072 50 43 29

info@edelsteinmassagen.de

www.edelstein-massagen.de/tuebingen

Cairn Elen Lebensschule Schwäbische Alb

Dagmar Fleck

Rossgumpenstrasse 10, 72336 Balingen-Zillhausen, Germany

Tel: +49 (0) 7435 91 99 32, Fax: +49 (0) 7435 91 99 31

info@cairn-elen.de, www.cairn-elen.de

Cairn Elen Lebensschule Odenwald

Franca Bauer, Berliner Strasse 1a, 64711 Erbach, Germany

Tel: +49 (0) 6062 91 97 62, Fax: +49 (0) 6062 91 97 63

info@cairn-elen.de, www.cairn-elen.de

Crystal Balance

Introductory courses, seminars, and training in Crystal Balance and other crystal massage, as well as dowsing courses, seminars and training in crystal healing.

Monika Grundmann

Bauhofstrasse 14, 91560 Heilsbronn, Germany
Tel: +49 (0) 9872 29 99, Fax: +49 (0) 9872 26 06, www.crystal-balance.com

Reflexology Zone Massage with Crystals

Institute, practise, lectures, seminars and training in reflexology zone therapy, including the use of crystal wands.

Ewald Kliegel

Rotenbergstrasse 154, 70190 Stuttgart, Germany
Tel: +49 (0) 172 712 48 89
info@reflex-zonen.de, www.reflex-zonen.de

More on Joya® massages, Joya® training and Joya® massage rollers can be found at www.joya.eu

More on crystal healing: www.crystalhealingbooks.com

Cairn Elen

'When Elen had ended her wanderings through the world, she set up a cairn at the end of Sarn Elen. Then her path turned back to the land between the evening and the morning. From this cairn are derived all stones that still stand at crossroads and that point the way.'*   *(from a Celtic legend)*

'Cairn Elen' – is the term used for the ancient stones set up at waysides in regions where the Gallic languages are spoken. They mark the spirit paths, as well as the earth energy paths and the paths of wisdom.

These paths are becoming increasingly forgotten. Just as the old paths of the earth are disappearing under modern asphalted roads, so much ancient knowledge too is disappearing under avalanches of data from modern knowledge and insights. The desire and the appeal of the Edition Cairn Elen is thus to preserve knowledge from ancient times and to re-connect it with modern insights – towards a flourishing future!

The Edition Cairn Elen of the Neue Erde Verlag is published by Michael Gienger. The goal of the Edition is to introduce hitherto unpublished knowledge from research and traditions. The emphasis is on nature, natural healing and health, as well as on awareness and spiritual freedom.

Stories, fairytales, novels, poetry and works of art, in addition to up-to-date specialist literature, are published within the framework of the Edition Cairn Elen. The knowledge passed on speaks not only to the intellect, but also to the heart of the reader.

Contact:

Edition Cairn Elen, Michael Gienger, Fürststraße 13, 72072 Tübingen, Germany. Tel. +49 (0) 7071 36 47 20, Fax: +49 (0) 7071 38 868
buecher@michael-gienger.de, www.michael-gienger.de

* Celt. 'cairn' = 'stone'; 'sarn' = 'path'; 'Elen, Helen' = 'goddess of the paths, roads'

Monika Grundmann
Crystal Balance
A step-by-step guide to beauty and health through crystal massage
Our physical wellbeing reflects every aspect of our lives and inner selves. As a result, massage is able to influence us on every level – mind, body and spirit.

The Crystal Balance method aims to help our bodies relax and recover, encouraging our soul and spirit to 'be themselves'. When we are truly 'ourselves', we are beautiful. It is as simple as that.
Paperback, full colour throughout, 112 pages, ISBN 978-1-84409-132-4

Ewald Kliegel
Crystal Wands
For healing, massage therapy and reflexology
What could you achieve with a crystal wand? How can you find out which crystal wand best suits your needs? How can you perform a relaxing massage combining crystal wands and reflexology? These are just a few of the questions answered in this practical guidebook. Learn to use crystal wands for reflexology, for massage, to trace meridian lines or to balance the chakras; whatever your therapeutic aim, these beautiful energetic tools can help you. Basic information on reflexology, crystal healing and testing methods is also included, as well as full massage programs for your immediate use.
Paperback, full colour, 144 pages, ISBN 978-1-84409-152-2

Michael Gienger
Crystal Massage for Health and Healing
This book introduces a spectrum of massage possibilities using healing crystals. The techniques have been developed and refined by experts, and this wisdom is conveyed in simple and direct language, enhanced by photos. Any interested amateur will be amazed at the wealth of new therapeutic possibilities that open up when employing the healing power of crystals.
112 Pages, full colour throughout, ISBN 978-1-84409-077-8

Michael Gienger
Gem Water
How to prepare and use more than 130 crystal waters for therapeutic treatments
Adding crystals to water is both visually appealing and healthy. It is a known fact that water carries mineral information and Gem Water provides effective remedies, acting quickly on a physical level. It is similar and complementary to wearing crystals, but the effects are not necessarily the same. Gem Water needs to be prepared and applied with care; this book explains everything you need to know to get started!
Paperback, 96 pages, ISBN 978-1-84409-131-7

Michael Gienger
Healing Crystals
The A - Z guide to 430 gemstones
All the important information about 430 healing gemstones in a neat pocket-book! Michael Gienger, known for his popular introductory work 'Crystal Power, Crystal Healing', here presents a comprehensive directory of all the gemstones currently in use. In a clear, concise and precise style, with pictures accompanying the text, the author describes the characteristics and healing functions of each crystal.
Paperback, 96 page, ISBN 978-1-84409-067-9

Michael Gienger
The Healing Crystals First Aid Manual
A practical A to Z of common ailments and illnesses and how they
can be best treated with Crystal Therapy
This is an easy-to-use A-Z guide for treating many common ailments and illnesses with the help of crystal therapy. It includes a comprehensive color appendix with photographs and short descriptions of each gemstone recommended.
288 pages, with 16 colour plates, ISBN 978-1-84409-084-6

Isabel Silveira
Quartz Crystals
A guide to identifying quartz crystals and their healing properties
This visually impressive book brings the reader up close to the beauty and diversity of the quartz crystal family. Its unique and concise presentation allows the reader to quickly and easily identify an array of quartz crystals and become familiar with their distinctive features and energetic properties.
Paperback, full colour throughout, 80 pages, ISBN 978-1-84409-148-5

Michael Gienger
Purifying Crystals
How to clear, charge and purify your healing crystals
The correct cleansing of healing crystals is an essential prerequisite for working with them successfully. But how can this be done effectively? There appear to be many different opinions on the subject. This useful little guidebook aims to provide the information needed about how many of the known methods work, and also clearly differentiates between the more and the less effective methods.
Paperback, full colour throughout, 64 pages, ISBN 978-1-84409-147-8

Joya – Crystal Massage for Everyone
First Edition 2009

This English edition
© 2009 Earthdancer GmbH
English translation © 2009 Astrid Mick

Editorial: Claudine Eleanor Bloomfield

Originally published in German as
Joya – Jeder kann massieren
World © Neue Erde GmbH, Saarbruecken, Germany
All rights reserved

Title page: photo Ines Blersch
    Design: Dragon Design UK Ltd.
Typesetting and graphics:
    Dragon Design UK Ltd.
Typeset in News Gothic

Entire production: Midas Printing
Printed and bound in China

ISBN 978-1-84409-168-3

Published by Earthdancer GmbH, an imprint of: Findhorn Press, 305a The Park, Findhorn, Forres, IV36 3TE, Great Britain
www.earthdancer.co.uk
www.findhornpress.com

EARTHDANCER A FINDHORN PRESS IMPRINT

For further information and book catalogue contact:
Findhorn Press, 305a The Park, Forres, IV36 3TE, Scotland.
Earthdancer Books is an imprint of Findhorn Press.
tel +44 (0)1309-690582, fax +44 (0)131 777 2711
info@findhornpress.com, www.earthdancer.co.uk, www.findhornpress.com

For more information on crystal healing visit www.crystalhealingbooks.com

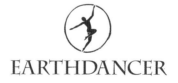

EARTHDANCER

A FINDHORN PRESS IMPRINT